DATE DUE

DEMCO

HEALTHCARE STRATEGY

STRATEGY

In Pursuit of Competitive Advantage

HEALTHCARE

STRATEGY

In Pursuit of Competitive Advantage

Roice D. Luke

Stephen L. Walston

Patrick Michael Plummer

AUPHA

HAP

Your board, staff, or clients may also benefit from this book's insight. For more information on quantity discounts, contact the Health Administration Press Marketing Manager at (312) 424-9470.

08   07   06   05   04   5   4   3   2   1

Library of Congress Cataloging-in-Publication Data

Luke, Roice D.
    Healthcare strategy: in pursuit of competitive advantage / Roice D. Luke, Stephen L. Walston, Patrick Michael Plummer.
        p. cm.
    Includes bibliographical references and index.
    ISBN 1-56793-215-0 (alk. paper)
    1. Medical policy—United States. 2. Health planning—United States. 3. Health care reform—United States. I. Walston, Stephen Lee. II. Plummer, Patrick Michael. III. Title.

    RA395.A3L84 2003
    362.1'0973—dc22   2003056608

The paper used in this publication meets the minimum requirements of American National Standard for Information Sciences—Permanence of Paper for Printed Library Materials, ANSI Z39.48-1984. ∞ ™

Project manager: Jane Williams; Acquisitions manager: Janet Davis; Layout editor: Amanda J. Karvelaitis; Cover designer: Trisha Lartz

Health Administration Press   Association of University Programs
A division of the Foundation of the   in Health Administration
    American College of Healthcare Executives   730 11th Street, NW
One North Franklin Street   4th Floor
Suite 1700   Washington, DC 20001
Chicago, IL 60606   (202) 638-1448
(312) 424-2800

Brief Contents

Detailed Contents

Preface

COMPETITION HAS BECOME a way of life in almost all healthcare markets. As a result, most healthcare organizations now actively engage in the pursuit of competitive advantage. As they do so, however, these competitors are forced to confront a number of important and distinctive realities. First, healthcare is highly unique in the sense that competitive advantage is heavily cloaked in institutional restraints, which stem from

- an extensive array of regulatory and payment structures,
- a highly restrictive and dynamic moral and religious milieu,
- high levels of interorganizational interdependencies among provider entities, and
- historically grounded expectations for autonomy by many health professional groups.

These and other factors, which are exclusive to this industry, shape and limit a healthcare organization's strategic choices to a degree not experienced in other industries. Therefore, application of strategy to healthcare must be filtered through the prism of industry- and organizational-level constraints.

Second, serious competition arrived in healthcare only recently; as a result, many healthcare organizations are fairly high on the strategy learning curve. Most importantly, many organizations are facing for the first time myriad challenges that accompany significant and rapid increases in organizational scale, combined with increasing threats from ever larger and more powerful competitors and buyers. Organizations today must be far more skillful in digesting and assimilating the many and diverse businesses acquired through mergers and acquisitions, identifying appropriate organizational forms to manage new organizational configurations, finding new funding sources, and balancing concomitant increases in market power with continuing obligations to serve the public interest.

Third, some imaginative organizational forms have emerged, which are often poorly understood by researchers and policymakers and even by those who have created them. These organizational arrangements range from full ownership types to loosely coupled alliance structures. The latter are especially notable because they typically retain many of the distinctive missions, power centers, administrative staffs, organizational structures, and service capacities of the joined provider entities. As a result, many of the newly formed systems are struggling to integrate and unify their combined operations.

Fourth, healthcare delivery and strategy formulation are still largely local, despite the significant restructuring that has occurred in recent years. In the turbulent 1990s, some of the largest and most far-flung healthcare organizations failed at sustaining national strategies and learned difficult lessons about the need to focus on local markets and competition. Thus, organizations that succeeded at competition tend to be those that have created strong local and, in a number of cases, regional positions. Importantly, strong local (and regional) positions serve to counter the growing power of managed care companies and threats from aggressive local rivals. Thus, healthcare organizations that are spread across multiple markets must engage in strategic combat on two fronts: one at the company level and the other within each of their local markets. Healthcare organizations must figure out how best to structure decision-making processes and authority between their corporate and local units.

Fifth, high levels of consolidation must be addressed by those who formulate strategy in the healthcare industry. Because of consolidation, the focus of strategy has to shift away from individual provider units and toward provider collectives. In the hospital sector, for example, focusing on single hospitals might have been appropriate prior to the 1990s. Today, given that so many hospitals are members of multihospital systems, a more collective view must be considered.

GUIDING CONCEPTS AND INNOVATIONS

Of all the administrative disciplines one can study in an academic or corporate classroom, strategy analysis is possibly the one most fully intertwined with the real world. It is a discipline that requires the analyst to have a clear understanding not only of the organizations seeking competitive advantage but also of the competitors, markets, and broader environments that surround those organizations. This point is even more necessary in the study of strategy in so unique an industry as healthcare.

In a teaching setting, the most common approach to bridging the worlds of academics and practice has been to apply the concepts and techniques of strategy analysis using a variety of historical cases. Such cases typically focus on decisions made by single organizations at distant points in time. Although this approach might have been acceptable in prior decades, it is not ideal today. This is especially true given the rapid turbulence and changes that are occurring in the external environment of healthcare and the fact that strategic information is now so accessible via the Internet. One can find on the web real-time data on strategic decisions, organizational objectives, finances, organizational configurations, organizational structures, competitor compositions and maneuvers, market conditions, environmental change, and so forth. The increasing availability of such information makes possible the comprehensive study of strategy almost at the same time as organizational and market changes happen. In effect, the web provides many "cases" to be studied.

This book takes advantage of the rich resources on the web. It is not cluttered by a collection of historical cases; rather, it provides contemporaneous examples of developments in the world of strategy, most of which can be followed up by searching information on the web. This book is accompanied by an innovative, web-based study system called *Strategy Resources*. Drawing on StratCenter, an extensive database of hospital systems and markets, the Strategy Resources allows for the study of systems and markets across the country. The national focus of StratCenter enables readers to compare systems to their rivals as well as to members of the same strategic groups—that is, competitors across the country that have similar strategic business models. Through StratCenter, markets may also be analyzed in depth and compared to their strategic market groups—that is, markets across the country that have similar market characteristics. To access the Strategy Resources, visit the Health Administration Press web site—http://www. ache.org/pubs/luke.cfm.

Included in the Strategy Resources is an online Instructor's Manual, which facilitates the use of StratCenter and the web as study tools. The Instructor's Manual provides definitions of key concepts; descriptions of data; and study questions and assignments, which range from examining mission statements to comparing market structures and competitors across markets.

With the web, the Strategy Resources exposes students of strategy to the major systems, markets, and strategic issues of the day. This broader, more comprehensive focus contrasts starkly with the restricted view of strategy when it is examined through a few historical cases.

Finally, the book avoids restating strategic generalities and formulas that might apply broadly to most industries but not necessarily to the healthcare industry. Instead, it selectively applies and adapts the concepts and methods of strategy analysis to the important features and realities of healthcare.

STRUCTURE OF THE BOOK

This book is organized around two central ideas:

1. The means of strategy are driven by the desired end of strategy—that is, competitive advantage.
2. Strategy is determined by the characteristics of individual organizations, the capabilities and behaviors of their competitors, and the structures of the markets within which they operate.

The book discusses five major sources of competitive advantage. Each of these sources begins with the letter P for ease of remembering them:

- Pace
- Position
- Potential
- Performance
- Power

In Chapter 1 ("The Concept of Strategy"), we look in on the current debate about the meaning of strategy. We resolve that debate, for our own purposes, by defining strategy in terms of competitive advantage. This conceptualization reflects the fact that healthcare has entered a highly competitive market environment in which organizations vie aggressively to gain advantage over their rivals. Chapter 2 ("Strategy Analysis Framework") lays out the conceptual foundations that are essential in analyzing strategy. It emphasizes the concepts and methods developed by industrial organization economists as well as by the advocates of the resource-based view of strategy. Together, these two perspectives turn our attention internally to the workings of organizations and externally to the opportunities and threats emanating from the markets and the broader environment. The chapter also presents the overall framework upon which the analysis of strategy in the book is based.

In Chapter 3 ("Strategic Intent"), the value context of strategy is presented. Specifically, we explore the "directional" strategies (mission, values, and vision) that provide a critical context in which healthcare organizations consider how (and whether) to grow and to engage in competitive battle. These directional strategies are especially important in the healthcare industry, given the powerful institutional context in which the industry provides services to the sick and vulnerable. Chapter 4 ("Market Structure") addresses one of the two key concepts in the book (the other is strategy and the associated sources of competitive advantage). In Chapter 2, the analysis of market structure is placed within a general framework. Chapter 4 moves beyond that framework, considering some of the ways markets are defined and market structure is measured. Also in this chapter, we introduce the concepts of strategic groups and strategic market groups. These groups provide essential ways to highlight the distinctive strategies and challenges facing organizations and markets. The assessment of market structure is especially important in analyzing strategy in markets that are dominated by a few powerful players, under which healthcare markets are increasingly typified.

Chapter 5 ("Pace Strategies") presents one of the more elusive sources of competitive advantage. Pace addresses the timing, aggressiveness, and other actions taken by organizations in pursuit of competitive advantage. All organizations engaged in market combat must consider when to move and with what type of intensity. Chapter 6 ("Position, Potential, and Performance Strategies") addresses three other sources of advantage. Position projects an organization's distinctive value to consumers. Potential states the organization's capabilities in acquiring sustainable internal resources and capabilities. Performance deals with the implementation of strategy. No strategy will be effective if it is not managed and carried out effectively.

Chapters 7 through 9 focus on the fifth source of competitive advantage—power. In general, power strategies produce advantages derived from the buildup of organizational mass, which results from expansions in the size and diversity of businesses run by an organization. Chapter 7 ("Power Strategies") discusses power as a general source of advantage.

Here, the important distinction between relative and absolute strategy is considered. Some organizations gain advantage primarily by being large generally, while others do so by being large relatively—that is, relative (by market share, for example) to other competitors within given markets. We also distinguish between corporate and business unit strategy, a distinction that has become increasingly important in recent years as healthcare organizations have become larger and more complex.

Chapter 8 ("Horizontal Expansion") examines the most common and, some might argue, the most important form of a power strategy. Horizontal expansion is the act of increasing organizational and market power by combining the size and number of same-sector business units. We distinguish horizontal strategies pursued at the company level from those pursued within individual markets. Of particular interest are differences in size and patterns of geographic configuration. For example, the approaches that widely dispersed organizations take to gain advantage differ greatly from those used by clustered, single-market or regional systems. Chapter 9 ("Vertical Integration") discusses the power strategy that became popular in the 1990s but that many healthcare organizations found difficult to implement. We emphasize some of the more important challenges inherent in vertical integration.

Chapter 10 ("Organizational Structure") explores one of the more difficult areas facing healthcare organizations: the design of an organizational structure that is compatible with an organization's values, expectations of primary stakeholders, and strategies. Organizational structure is especially demanding in healthcare, given the diversity of large and complex healthcare organizations. Also, institutional constraints limit the range and effectiveness of options available for structuring organizations in healthcare. Because of its internal focus, organizational structure fits best within two sources of competitive advantage—potential and performance.

ACKNOWLEDGMENT

We would like to thank the following companies that funded the Williamson Institute in its study of markets and systems across the country. Over a six-year period in the mid-1990s, these companies supported data collection and a series of site visits to major markets. Interviews were conducted with heads of the leading competitors in those markets.

- McKesson Corporation, beginning with General Medical Corporation, which was acquired by McKesson in the course of the study;

- Johnson & Johnson;
- EDS; and
- DuPont.

Roice D. Luke, PH.D.
Professor and Chair
Department of Health Administration
Virginia Commonwealth University

Stephen L. Walston, PH.D.
Associate Professor
Master in Health Administration Program
Indiana University

Patrick Michael Plummer
Founder and CEO
myHealthcareNews.com

PART I

Concepts and Context

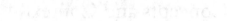

Chapter 1

The Concept of Strategy

...tactics teaches the use of the armed forces in engagements, and strategy the use of engagements to attain the object of the war.

—*Clausewitz (2000, 330)*

STRATEGY IS THE central concept in strategy analysis. Although this statement might seem so obvious, it tells the student of strategy that the field of business strategy is still somewhat unresolved on what strategy actually is. A number of reasons contribute to this complexity. First, the field represents the convergence of multiple disciplines, including economics, organization theory, general business, marketing, finance, and geography (to name but a few). As a result, strategy is often viewed through different lenses, depending on one's background and purpose. Second, and perhaps more important, business strategy is a very young field. As a result, not all of the concepts and approaches to analysis are yet well established or agreed on. Significantly, the field of healthcare strategy is even less well developed, arriving in healthcare only in the past decade. Consequently, we have much to learn about how strategy should be applied in so distinctive and important an industry as healthcare.

Because of its centrality to analysis, we devote this introductory chapter to defining strategy, which we do in several steps. First, we trace the evolution of the concept, both generally and specifically, as it applies to healthcare. Second, we discuss the debate currently swirling around the concept and offer a resolution so that we can move on to analysis. The resolution comes by defining strategy in terms of the pursuit of competitive advantage, and this resolution is consistent with where the field appears to be headed at the present time. Third, we introduce the major sources of competitive advantage that most organizations use in their strategic maneuvering. Ironically, a debate also brews about the preferred source of competitive advantage. We take no side in this debate. However, we believe that any of the identified sources is acceptable so long as it produces the end result of strategy—competitive advantage.

THE EVOLUTION OF STRATEGY

The concept of business strategy can be traced very far back in history to many situations, including the context of war (Bracker 1980; Chandler 1977; Fahey and Christensen 1986; Huff and Reger 1987; McCraw 1998; McKiernan 1997; Miller and Cardinal 1994; Mintzberg 1994; Prahalad and Hamel 1994; Schendel and Hoffer Schendel 1979). Strategy in war is obviously important, given the decisive role it plays in shaping the outcomes of battle. As Clausewitz (2000, 390) put it, "Strategy…[gives] an aim to the whole…. [It] maps out the plan of the war, and to the aforesaid aim it affixes the series of acts which lead to [the object of war]." This quotation echoes the central purpose of strategy—to provide the blueprint by which the end can be attained under conditions of direct combat. This is true whether the "war" is actual military conflict or market competition.

Just as the significance of strategy rises with the threat of war, so too does the import of business strategy when rivalry intensifies. From the Middle Ages through the nineteenth century, small entrepreneurs or loosely organized craft guilds comprised most business entities. Their attention was more directed to keeping outsiders from entering their territories than to gaining advantages over nearby rivals. For the most part, they were too small to influence the behaviors of other local businesses. When large, often monopolistic enterprises emerged, their focus tended to center on global threats and on how the levers of governmental and military power might be used to further business objectives. With the industrial and political revolutions of the late nineteenth century through the early twentieth century, the markets in the western world underwent significant changes in both structure and behavior. Modern transportation, manufacturing techniques, and various mechanical and electronic inventions all led to the formation of many large business organizations and the evolution of increasingly aggressive markets. Large, vertically integrated, conglomerate firms emerged, as did many small- and medium-sized businesses. Thus, upon entering the twentieth century, as Pankaj Ghemawat (2000, 3) put it, "Adam Smith's 'invisible hand' came to be supplemented by what Alfred D. Chandler, Jr., a famous (Harvard) historian, has termed the 'visible' hand of professional managers."

Price has always been a central focus of competition, although as firms got larger and larger, fears of competition-driven, downwardly spiraling prices led many rivals to seek other nonprice ways by which to compete. Out of this bog of combative posturing and maneuvering among powerful rivals came the modern form of competitive strategy.

Economists attempted to express the visible hand in a variety of ways, most prominently in the formulations of oligopolistic and monopolistic competitive market models (Coase 1937; Penrose 1959; Shumpeter 1942). Unfortunately, these models tended toward abstraction and public policy applications and shed limited light on the problem of deciding business strategy. Interestingly, even though the concepts and techniques of strategy analysis were fairly well established by the latter half of the 1900s, not until the 1980s (see Porter 1980 for example) were the models and concepts of economics translated in terms that made them easily accessible to strategy analysts, which is a point discussed further below and in subsequent chapters.

Strategy thus became a primary concern for business managers at that time in history when competitors gained sufficient market power to be capable of affecting the prospects of their rivals, which, for the most part, occurred well within the twentieth century. The true importance of strategy then is observed during conditions of combat and competitive threat within markets. Although strategy is certainly applicable when threats emanate from the more general environment, strategy analysts earn their stripes in circumstances in which rivals contest head to head. This is the fertile ground of strategy, the point-counterpoint of market competition.

Strategy Comes to Healthcare

Strategy arrived more recently in healthcare than it did in most other industries. As occurred in the business world generally, heightened market threat initiated healthcare's shift to a strategic orientation. By contrast to general business, however, the shift took place within a very short span of time, although precipitating factors had bubbled beneath the surface for many years. This rapid movement of strategy into healthcare explains in part the turbulence in strategy concept and approach that plagues healthcare today.

From the 1960s on, a variety of factors in healthcare and the general environment produced powerful pressures for change, including especially a more market-oriented economy in healthcare. Despite growing pressures, healthcare lingered on the margins of serious market competition for several decades. Deeply embedded in institutional values and historically sanctioned community missions, healthcare organizations remained fairly well buffered against increasing competitive threats. What other industries called "markets" healthcare referred to as "systems" (as in the healthcare system). This difference in terminology reflects the cooperative, as opposed to competitive, interrelationships that healthcare providers have been expected to establish with one another. Providers historically have served a kind of public function, regardless of whether they were organized as public, not-for-profit, or for-profit entities. Before the 1990s, the vast majority of organizations in healthcare tended to be singular entities composed mostly of individual physician groups, hospitals, state or regional insurance companies, and so forth.

With healthcare costs spiraling out of control beginning in the mid-1960s, local governments sought ways to stave off the unrelenting increases. In the 1970s and 1980s, the federal government attempted to regulate healthcare providers, implicitly retaining the assumption that market competition might not provide the appropriate remedy given the peculiarities of the industry. Then came the managed competition revolution of the 1990s, with its emphasis on countervailing buyer power and competition in both managed care and provider markets. This was a revolution both because of the breathtaking pace in which change occurred and because of the readiness with which the industry and nation seemed willing to adopt market and payment incentives as the preferred mechanisms for curing the industry's ills. Consequently, in just a few short years, healthcare transformed itself from a sleepy community service system to a dynamic, market-driven industry. As a result, strategy became a primary basis on which many healthcare organizations now plot their futures.

Chain Reactions to Managed Care

The spark that ignited the change, if one can be isolated from all other determinants, had to have been the chorus of concern from both private and public sectors directed at rising costs. Many large firms and government entities threatened to use their individual buying power to shop and negotiate for more favorable prices on insurance premiums. Many private firms, most of which were large- and medium-sized businesses, endeavored to form into business coalitions, thereby threatening to consolidate their buying power still further. At the same time, the federal government attempted to convert the delivery of Medicare and Medicaid services into managed care formats, adding an even larger price-focused buyer to the mix—the government.

Much of the fulmination that occurred did not translate directly into effective market action. The business coalitions, for example, were a notable disappointment (Bodenheimer and Sullivan 1998); they were unable to hold their coalitions together or to convert them into price-negotiating entities. Various state and federal government experiments failed to achieve their promise. The primary result of all of these changes, however ineffective in the end, was that they raised expectations to such a level that the healthcare industry quickly readied itself for a new era of market competition.

The first wave of responses included insurance companies transforming themselves into managed care organizations, aggressively seeking to enter new markets, and pursuing merger and acquisition targets. Healthcare providers also became involved by becoming larger organizational entities in which economics—that is, strategy—played a vital role in determining the direction and ultimate survival of the organization. Many hospitals became members of multihospital systems, largely driven by a desire to join up with one of the many locally forming strategic hospital alliances. Even physicians got into the act, although overall they were less successful than hospitals or managed care companies in consolidating their markets. Nevertheless, many joined large physician groups, whether owned by physicians, hospitals, or physician practice management companies. Concurrently, traditional attachments to communities and missions began to erode and voluntary contributions played increasingly more marginal roles in funding healthcare provider organizations.

Members of the supply channel were also caught up in the merger and acquisition frenzy. Increasingly threatened by the growing power of providers and managed care companies and the already well established power of many very large pharmaceutical and medical supply companies, distribution companies aggressively pursued mergers and acquisitions within their own sector. They combined both within and across product sectors (medical/surgical, pharmaceutical, and home health), producing by the end of the 1990s a small number of dominating distributors vying to control the supply channel.

Unknown Factors of Strategy in Healthcare

Within just a few years (mostly in the 1990s), many payer, provider, and distribution markets consolidated. As a result, strategy became an even more important tool by which healthcare organizations adapt to uncertain market environments. However, given the relative recentness of this development, much can still be learned about the applications of strategy in the healthcare industry. We have yet to determine, for example, how the evolving clinical and information technologies will shape the markets and restructure delivery systems. We need to ascertain whether or not the highly touted integrated systems model will become the strategic ideal for healthcare organization; in the 1990s, most industry insiders assumed it would do just that (American Hospital Association 1990, 1992; Catholic Health Association 1992; Conrad and Shortell 1996; The Advisory Board 1993). Also, we do not know what directions provider consolidation will take in the future, as healthcare organizations experiment with organizational power as an instrument of market competition. We do not know how the increased rivalry will affect the historic willingness of healthcare providers to cooperate at the local market level.

From a public policy point of view, we do not know whether the market experiment will work in meeting the three objectives of containing costs, enhancing quality, and improving access to care. We also do not know how the new market environment will affect the innovativeness that has so characterized the U.S. healthcare system. Perhaps more importantly, we do not yet know where the moral and ethical lines will be drawn, as entities that were historically entrusted with the mission of healing the sick engage in mortal combat with one another.

Clearly, the stakes are very high. No doubt the public will be watching to see whether the new competitive models in healthcare will serve the collective interest in the end. Healthcare has entered some very interesting and uncharted waters as it attempts to apply traditional business models and objectives in the context of a highly institutionalized environment. Nonetheless, within this environment is where healthcare strategists ply their profession, the concepts and techniques for which are the focus of this book.

Lessons for Strategy Analysis

Two key points can be drawn from the foregoing discussion. First, strategy is a relative concept. It is pursued largely as a counter response to the actual and expected actions and capabilities of rivals. More specifically, strategy specifies the ways that competitors hope to gain advantage over one another. Second, approaches to gaining advantage can only be deduced by examining the variety of factors that together shape the means and intensity by which competitors react to perceived market threats. These factors can be summarized in numerous ways:

- Broader environment
- Market structure
- Conduct/behaviors of rivals
- Internal competencies of one's organization and of competitors

Each of these factors places conditions on the degree to which and the ways by which organizations pursue and ultimately gain advantage.

Concerned about a decline in federal funding (an indicator stemming from the broader environment factor), one organization might focus on internal efficiencies as the best way to ensure that it will have sufficient resources to compete effectively. Another, confronted by increasing concentration among buyers (a market structure factor), might seek merger opportunities to countervail expected buyer threats. Still another, anticipating an attempt on the part of a major rival to strengthen its position in a particular service area (a competitor response factor), might act preemptively by expanding rapidly into that same service area. Perceiving its greatest asset to be its management capabilities (internal competency factor), a competitor might build on that strength by investing heavily in information technologies.

These factors constitute the analytic grist of strategy analysis. They are the ingredients most likely to be considered by an organization when deciding how to gain advantage or when evaluating a strategy. Most competitors will investigate all four of these but might find only one or two to be particularly pertinent to their choice of strategy. These factors are discussed in detail in Chapter 2.

CONCEPT IN SEARCH OF A DEFINITION

Strategic thinking and analysis require a clear understanding of the concept of strategy. However, such a simple truth has not always been appreciated in the field of strategy. In fact, only a little over 20 years ago authors Schendel and Hoffer Schendel (1979) proclaimed strategy to be the centerpiece of strategic management:

> Today the policy field is in need of a **new paradigm** that can end the continual and pointless redefinition of concepts used in both practice and teaching…. The new paradigm we propose…is that of 'strategic management,' and it rests squarely on the concept of strategy.

Few would question the centrality of the concept of strategy to market competition today. Yet, the "continual and pointless redefinition of concepts" reflects an ongoing frustration many have with the seeming aimlessness with which the concept has been defined over the years. Table 1.1 presents some of the diversity of views that have evolved over the past 40 years, ranging in terminology from "policies" to "patterns." Faced with this uncertainty of concept, Henry Mintzberg (1994, 23–29) offered not one but five conceptual equivalents of strategy, perhaps hoping that in so doing he could at least encircle the elusive concept:

1. Plan: a guide or course of action into the future
2. Ploy: a specific maneuver intended to outwit an opponent or competitor
3. Position: determination of particular products in particular markets
4. Perspective: an organization's way of doing things
5. Pattern: consistency in behavior over time

The field has moved beyond defining strategy as a formal "plan" (as Mintzberg concluded as well). Strategy may be the centerpiece or the object of a plan, but it is not a plan per se. A "ploy" may appear somewhat synonymous with strategy, but it is a narrower concept that perhaps corresponds more with tactics than with strategy. "Perspective" is an interesting concept. As used by Mintzberg, the term refers broadly to a firm's overall purposes and focus. As such, closely associating perspective with missions and values (discussed in Chapter 3) seems more appropriate than listing it as a possible definition of strategy.

Another concept offered by Mintzberg is "position," which is closest to being a major constituent of strategy. Established market positions represent organizations' successful efforts to imbue their products with distinctive value and embed that value in the minds of consumers. If they

Table 1.1. Some Definitions of Strategy Over Time

- Determinator of the basic long-run goals (Chandler 1962)
- Rule for making decisions determined by product/market scope (Ansoff 1965)
- Unified, comprehensive, and integrated plan (Glueck 1976)
- What business strategy is all about is, in a word, competitive advantage (Ohmae 1983)
- Plan...ploy...pattern...position...perspective (Mintzberg, Ahlstrand, and Lampel 1998)
- Pattern of decisions an organization makes (Hax 1990)
- Positioning a business to maximize the value of capabilities to distinguish it from its competitors (Porter 1980)

Sources: Ansoff, H. I. 1965. *Corporate Strategy: An Analytic Approach to Business Policy for Growth and Expansion*. New York: McGraw-Hill; Chandler, A. D. 1962. *Strategy and Structure: Chapters in the History of the Industrial Enterprise*. Cambridge, MA: MIT Press; Gluck, F. W. 1976. *Business Policy: Strategy Formulation and Management Action*, 2nd ed. New York: McGraw-Hill; Hax, A. C. 1990. "Redefining the Concept of Strategy and the Strategy Formation Process." *Planning Review* 18 (3): 34–40; Mintzberg, H., B. Ahlstrand, and J. Lampel. 1998. *Strategy Safari: A Guided Tour Through the Wilds of Strategic Management*. New York: Simon & Schuster; Ohmae, K. 1983. *Mind of the Strategist: Business Planning for a Corporate Advantage*. New York: Viking Penguin; Porter, M. E. 1980. *Competitive Strategy: Techniques for Analyzing Industries and Competitors*. New York: The Free Press.

are successful in achieving distinctiveness and that position indeed is perceived to have value, then the position will likely generate competitive advantage and serve the interests of strategy. On the other hand, efforts to restrict the definition of strategy to positioning have generated considerable debate, which we discuss later when we examine the sources of competitive advantage.

The fifth conceptualization of strategy offered by Mintzberg is "pattern." Here, Mintzberg addresses an important aspect of strategy formulation—that it is more the product of organizational learning than a one-time decision. Although insights into the processes and patterns of organizational learning are helpful and important (see Strategy Note 1.1), they provide little direction to the actual meaning of strategy. Processes are just that—processes. They represent the steps through which strategies pass as they move from great ideas to seasoned implementation. They do not constitute the essence of the concept itself. Despite this, however,

STRATEGY NOTE 1.1. MINTZBERG'S CONCEPTS OF PATTERN AND ORGANIZATIONAL LEARNING

The emphasis on strategy as pattern flows directly from Mintzberg's groundbreaking research into the role that organizational learning plays in strategy formulation. We comment on this theory not because we consider pattern to be an appropriate definition of strategy (which we do not) but because of the valuable insights the analysis of patterns provides in the practice of strategy formulation.

Figure 1A presents Mintzberg's scheme for conceptualizing strategy as a process or a pattern. Having studied the stages through which organizations pass in formulating strategy, Mintzberg concluded that *realized* strategies—those that actually come into being—do not always resemble the often-imposing *intended* strategies, which are commonly thought to be the product of executive visioning. On the way to strategy implementation, however, new insights, changes in the environment, added market intelligence, and other factors weigh in. As a result, strategies often evolve and change over time. They move from explicit and dramatic early formulations to refined conceptualizations that ultimately are implemented.

One can argue that many new insights picked up along the way represent mere tactical modifications of an original intended strategy. On the other hand, as Mintzberg recognized, sharp distinctions between tactics and strategies are not easily drawn:

> Strategies refer to the important things, tactics to the mere details…. But the very meaning of emergent strategy is that one can never be sure in advance which will prove to be which. In other words, mere details can eventually prove to be strategic. After all, as was pointed out in that old nursery rhyme, the war could well have been lost all for want of a nail in the shoe of a horse.

Others have confirmed Mintzberg's view of strategy as the product of an evolutionary process of formulation and implementation. In an earlier study, for example, Milton Leontiades (1980) observed that many *Fortune* 500 companies were far more cautious in implementing strategies than many believed. Rather than moving aggressively forward with some explicit strategic idea,

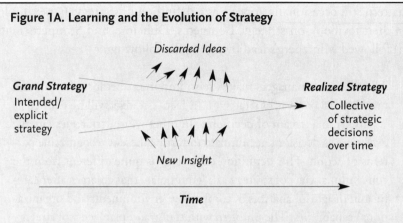

Figure 1A. Learning and the Evolution of Strategy

Discarded Ideas

Grand Strategy
Intended/
explicit
strategy

Realized Strategy
Collective
of strategic
decisions
over time

New Insight

Time

Source: Adapted with the permission of The Free Press, a Division of Simon & Schuster Adult Publishing Group, from THE RISE AND FALL OF STRATEGIC PLANNING: Reconceiving Roles for Planning, Plans, Planners by Henry Mintzberg. Copyright © 1994 by Henry Mintzberg.

organizations commonly implement strategies in small steps, taking care to be sure that each move merited the costly investments that are required. Leontiades characterized this as a kind of "incrementalism," thereby drawing a stark contrast between the visionary, even theatrical caricature of strategic decision making and the realities of how such decisions are made in the real world.

Because many strategic visions promise quite significant transformations of organizations, intended strategies often take on a kind of magnetic and mystical aura. Also, because they commonly come from the minds and visioning of organizational leaders, intended strategies readily assume an importance, exceeding what might otherwise be deduced from careful analyses of changing markets.

Strategy deals with the future, which is fraught with uncertainty and unpredictability. Caution, incrementalism, learning, and adaptability (as opposed to vision, courage, unswerving commitments, and boldness) thus become the hallmarks of strategy making in the real world. This does not mean that big ideas are not needed or important; rather, it means that the strategist must be fully aware that implemented strategy is often the product of much effort; changing assumptions about the environment; evolving technologies and demographics; limitations of existing resources and capabilities; market constraints; and, yes, more than a little serendipity.

pattern still occasionally appears as a definition of strategy. For example, in their textbook on strategy, Bourgeois, Duhaime, and Stimpert (1999, 11) followed Mintzberg's lead by saying the following:

> The decisions managers make are so important because they are the raw material or basis of strategies. In fact…strategy will be defined as 'a pattern in a stream of decisions.' In other words, strategies emerge over time as decisions accumulate to form coherent recognizable patterns of action. This definition of strategy is quite different from the conventional view of strategy as a 'grand plan' that emerges after careful and insightful analyses of competitive environments and organizational capabilities. The problem with the 'grand plan' view of strategy is that it does not reflect how strategies are actually formulated and implemented in most organizations.

As discussed in Strategy Note 1.1, viewing strategy simply as a "grand plan"—an overarching, never-to-be-altered plan of action—might be inappropriate. A strategy can be grand once implemented, but the original visions might or might not remain standing by the time the strategy decision and implementation processes are completed. That said, labeling strategy as a process, as a series of decisions, or as a pattern begs the question of what it is. One resolution to this definition difficulty is to avoid defining the concept at all and to simply emphasize analytic techniques. This was the tack taken by Ghemawat (2000, ix) in his textbook *Strategy and the Business Landscape: Core Concepts*:

> Despite thoughtful attempts over the decades to define "strategy"…a rash of manifestos continue to emerge that purport to redefine the term. It would therefore be idiosyncratic to begin by tossing another definition onto the pile.

Ghemawat did not toss another definition onto the pile; instead, he pressed forward without conceptualizing the central focus of his book! Others have been less timid. Although, in accord with Ghemawat's concern, they have unwittingly and unhelpfully added to the growing pile.

Defining Strategy

The etymology of the term *strategy* is often traced to the Greek term for generalship— strategia (Merriam-Webster 2002)—which again returns us to the military context; in fact, most dictionary definitions begin with a phrase such as "the art and science of military." Other definitions state that strategy is a *means* to a specific *end*—for example, "a plan, method, or series of actions designed to achieve a specific goal or effect" (Wordsmyth 2002). Fortunately, despite residual wrangling over the concept, the field of business strategy appears to have come to the same conclusion: strategy specifies a means to a critically important end. This is a far better approach than defining strategy in terms of administrative byproducts (published plans), procedures (patterns), or organizational rules (policies). Significantly, the field also appears to have reached a consensus on the primary *end* of strategy: to attain *competitive advantage* in the marketplace (see Barney 1991; Gluck, Kaufman, and Steven 1980; Montgomery and Porter 1991; Porter 1985). This end is achieved through some means, which in effect are the intended and/or realized strategies of organizations. This leads us to a means-end definition: Strategies are those key concepts and ideas that organizations use (or have used) to achieve and sustain competitive advantage over their rivals.

However this definition is worded or phrased, it clearly captures those ideas that lead organizations toward increased competitive advantage. We have selected the above definition purposefully, and our reasons are discussed in the following sections.

As Concepts and Ideas

In strategy formulation, the means and ends of strategy are for the most part conceptual. They are the ideas leaders associate with how they hope to win at competition. These ideas become the logical bases for marshalling an organization's resources and for focusing the attention of its members on the goal of gaining advantage. Such ideas might lead an organization to commit itself to making dramatic moves, such as engaging in merger and acquisition activities to build market share and, possibly, market dominance. In this case, merger would be the intended means to achieve the end of market dominance.

The means of strategy need not always involve major commitments of new resources. An organization can conclude, for example, that it already has attained a considerable advantage in the market; therefore, its strategic idea might be to hold the line, stay the course, and emphasize mere refinements of what that organization is currently doing. In this case, the means is to stick to the knitting (so to speak) and the end to sustain established market advantages. In sum, whatever an organization conceives as its basis for attaining and sustaining advantage becomes the essence of the organization's strategy. As to what specifically should be considered the means of strategy, we point out that residual arguments remain about which particular sources of advantage are better or more appropriate, a debate we discuss and seek to resolve in this chapter.

As Mintzberg (1994) noted, many organizations express ideas about strategy as "intended" or broad, overarching conceptualizations of how they hope to gain advantage in the marketplace. The problem with this, as discussed in Strategy Note 1.1, is such ideas often assume a level of un-merited strategic importance and, as a consequence, organizations become overly committed to them. Strategic visions easily present simplistic; immutable; and, therefore, distorted views of reality that are problematic when the environment is turbulent and uncertain, which was the case for healthcare in the 1990s, for example. However, the need for organizational learning does erode the need for intellectual constructs to guide and give impetus to strategic action and to rally organizational members in pursuit of a common cause, even if those ideas are big. Grand visions can and often do play crucial roles in overcoming organizational inertia and thus in facilitating change. Organizations can benefit immensely by formulating summative and even grand strategic ideas. Nevertheless, they do need to be adaptable and act incrementally as they move toward strategy implementation. Grand ideas are fine, even desirable, so long as they are not too grand or fixed given the circumstances.

As Past and Future Actions

Strategy is more than the sum of new ideas that point to future actions and investments. It includes also the cumulative effects of past actions and investments in capabilities, resources, positions, acquisitions, and so forth, at least to the extent that such contribute to competitive advantage. By melding together past with future decisions and investments, strategies become eminently integrative. Following is an example of this concept.

The strategies pursued by Food Lion, a large grocery store chain, illustrate how past and future strategic actions are interrelated, comprising the company's overall strategy. Food Lion continues to assess new markets or ways by which to increase market shares. At the same time, all acquisition and entry decisions are guided by Food Lion's long-established strategy of building and maintaining low-cost positions. This position, however, is the product of years of investment in personnel, facilities, advertising, management and control systems, and so forth. These past decisions and investments cumulatively add up to the advantage currently

STRATEGY NOTE 1.2. THE CASE OF FOOD LION: USING STRATEGIES OR TACTICS?

The Food Lion case raises that important distinction between strategy and tactics we have already discussed. A number of Food Lion's approaches to gaining advantage might seem more tactical (e.g., attaining efficiencies in the distribution and the handling and storage of products) than strategic. One organization's tactics, however, might be another's strategies. An organization that is deeply involved in a merger with a rival might consider strategy execution to be tactical, while another might view implementation as highly strategic given that success with implementation can make the difference between success and failure.

Implementation as strategy (or as a tactic, depending on the role it plays in producing competitive advantage) was especially important in the 1990s for those hospitals that attempted to combine into loosely coupled delivery systems. Many had hoped that such loose forms would facilitate the accomplishment of major strategic objectives while preserving cherished organizational autonomies. Because they had to compete against tightly coupled, ownership-based systems, competitors formed as loose arrangements found that implementation was critical to strategic success. Much, therefore, depended on the amount of power they needed to delegate to the collective's center, the mechanisms created to coordinate the otherwise autonomous partners, and the inherent trust each side had in the other (Powell 1990). Failure to deal successfully with matters of structuring and coordination meant the demise of these partnerships. They could not, therefore, relegate implementation to the category of mere tactical details.

attained by Food Lion. Food Lion's strategy thus combines past decisions and investments with future decisions and thinking about how best to maintain and expand the company's competitive advantage. (See Strategy Note 1.2.)

As a Tool for Achieving and Sustaining Advantage

As discussed in Chapter 5, merely gaining an advantage is often insufficient in this world of rapid change (D'Aveni 1994). Competitors will not likely sit on the sidelines while their rivals maneuver to gain advantage. Rather, they will actively search for ways to imitate or indirectly counter and erode any advantages attained (or hoped to be attained) by their rivals. Rapid technological advance, shifting economics, increasingly mobile and demanding populations, and unpredictable changes in consumer tastes all reinforce the importance of adaptation and change.

Competitive advantages are, as a result, sometimes elusive and temporary. They are not just attained. Strategists must contemplate possible reactions and subsequent second-order and third-order steps that might need to be taken. In other words, strategies must meet the dual tests of advantage and sustainability, both of which are required for a strategy to be successful over time. (Sustainability is discussed further in chapters 2 and 6.)

COMPETITIVE ADVANTAGE

Before considering the sources of competitive advantage, the concept of advantage is first defined: Competitive advantage accrues to an organization when it experiences an increase in market power as a result of the actions it has taken, capabilities or resources it has attained, or benefits it has gained.

It is common to consider as prima facie evidence of the presence of market power the fact that competitors are able to charge higher prices than might be expected in competitive markets (Scherer and Ross 1990). When applied to strategy, however, the indicators of market power are far broader. They include all evidence that competitors are able to influence the market behaviors (price or nonprice) of rivals, buyers, suppliers, substitutes, potential entrants, and other key market actors (Porter 1980).

A competitor that has achieved some spatial or product differentiation, for example, has in effect increased its ability to resist the threats of rivals. It has gained market power or, in our terms, increased its competitive advantage. Large organizational mass, high market shares, greater strategic mobility, financial war chests, great management systems, competent management and clinical staff, and many other sources of advantage all produce market power and, accordingly, boost competitive advantage. They all are the primary focal points or the means of strategy.

The Debate Over the Sources of Competitive Advantage

The sources of *competitive advantage* fall within the Holy Grail of strategy analysis. These are the competencies, schemes, contrivances, stratagems, and even subtle and often proprietary insights or visions of organizational leaders that make advantage attainable. In sum, they are the means to the end of strategy. Competitive advantage and its sources thus represent two sides of the same coin; they cannot be separated.

One might think, therefore, that any and all sources of advantage, regardless of whether their effects are direct or indirect, fall within the domain of strategy. Yet, the business strategy field still actively debates the strategic correctness of one source over another. The resultant polemical posturing often degenerates into a rather unproductive ideological tug of war over favored sources (see Porter 1996; Barney 1991; Grant 1991; Eisenhardt and Martin 2000; Foss 1999). Despite this, a number of new and helpful insights into strategy have emerged.

Two sides have achieved the most prominence in the debate. On one side are those who stress certain external advantages—the advantages of attaining distinctive positions in the marketplace. After all, this side argues, does not everything come down to whether or not an organization's products are sufficiently distinctive that they sell more readily than do products of rivals? On the other side are those who focus on the *internal capabilities and resources* of organizations. This other side suggests that organizations win over time if they can sustain competencies that are both distinctive and valuable competitively. We argue that both sources are relevant, to the extent that they contribute to the end of competitive advantage. Moreover, they are highly interdependent. Internal factors contribute to the development of external advantages. *External positions* (and other advantages) enhance the degree to which organizations are able to build up internal competencies. They all constitute the raw materials from which the strategy analyst creates competitive advantage.

External Argument: Positioning

Michael Porter, a professor at the Harvard Business School and a noted expert on competitive strategy, is the most recognized figure to promote external *positioning*, which he considers to be the central focus of strategy. Porter (1980, 47) defined strategy as "...positioning a business to maximize the value of the capabilities that distinguish it from its competitors."

Porter recognizes that the end is to distinguish a business from its rivals—that is, to gain advantage over that rival; he also suggests that one way to do this is to gain a superior position in the marketplace. Porter identified two fundamental options that are most likely to generate advantage: low cost and high differentiation. He actually identified three generic strategies, the third of which is focus; focus is essentially a targeted version of the first two. (We discuss generic strategies further in Chapter 6.)

Porter (1996) has been unrelenting in his arguments on behalf of positioning. Ironically, in his highly influential book on competitive strategy, Porter (1980) discussed other ways (in addition to positioning) by which firms gain advantage over rivals. These included such well-recognized strategic maneuvers as building organizational mass to countervail buyers, sellers, and rivals; building switching costs; and erecting entry barriers. In his 1985 book, he turned inward and focused almost exclusively on internal activities of organizations that affect their success in implementing positioning strategies and that lead to gains in competitive advantage.

In an interesting variation on the Porter theme, Ginter, Swayne, and Duncan (2002, 14) coupled Porter's emphasis on positioning to Mintzberg's concept of *pattern*, producing the following composite definition:

> ...a strategy may be viewed as a behavioral pattern [Mintzberg's concept] that emerges from a stream of decisions concerning the positioning [Porter's concept] of the organization within its environment. In other words, when a sequence of decisions relating the organization to its environment exhibits a logical consistency [their concept], over time, a strategy will have been formed.

The joining of positioning and pattern is an apparent attempt to broaden the definition beyond Porter's unnecessarily limited construction. But does linking a nondefinition (pattern) to one that is too narrowly constructed (positioning) really add anything to our understanding of the concept? The addition of "logical consistency" to the mix seems designed to extract the concept from the tangle of Mintzberg's process definition. In the end, the combining of pattern with positioning and with logical consistency serves only to compound the problem of conceptualizing strategy.

Internal Argument: Capabilities and Resources

A strong counter to Porter's restrictive emphasis on positioning is known as the *resource-based view*. Adherents to this perspective argue that the internal elements of organizations—their unique and defensible capabilities and resources—are the primary means by which advantage is gained. Competitive advantage, they suggest, accrues to the organization that is better able to compete, not to the one that has attained a better position. If properly chosen, distinctive and valuable internal competencies enable firms to fight off imitation and substitution threats (see Chapter 6) and thus to win repeated market battles over time. The goal is to win the war, not just an isolated fight or two, which they imply is all that positioning achieves. Advantage is thus tied to an established base of strength if it can be sustained over time.

Advantage by Any Means Is Advantage

So which source of competitive advantage is the correct one—distinctive positioning or superior internal competencies? As one might expect, the answer is both. Unfortunately, organizations that emphasized internal strengths fell into the same trap as did Porter; they focused too restrictively on a single source of competitive advantage, overlooking the many other viable sources of advantage universally pursued by other organizations.

Advantage is the objective, regardless of its means or sources. One organization might gain an advantage by pursuing economies of scale, and another by focusing on achieving market dominance through acquisitions and merger. Still another might gain advantage by providing higher-quality products, and another by focusing on internal efficiencies and competencies. Others might employ all of these methods and more in the pursuit of competitive advantage. Conceptually, does it matter what the source of advantage is so long as it works, can be sustained, and is legal and ethical?

Organizations commonly work on more than one source at a time. The weights organizations give to any one source will be shaped by the key ideas they have adopted for how advantage might be attained. They will be conditioned by the specifics of an organization's situation—its capabilities, distinctive market structures, competitor advantages and moves, and, certainly, time.

THE SOURCES OF COMPETITIVE ADVANTAGE

There are as many sources of advantage as there are markets or competitors. Those sources can be grouped into categories for the purpose of studying them. To summarize the various sources, we adopt the typology identified by Luke, Begun, and Walston (2000). They reduced all of the sources to five general categories, which are all labeled with P for ease of remembering:

Source	Basis for Advantage
Pace	Measured timing and intensity of strategic action

Figure 1.1. The Five Major Sources of Competitive Advantage

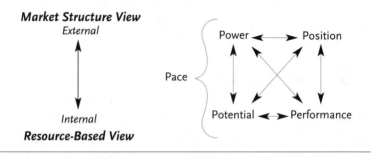

Position	Projection of distinctive and valued images to consumers
Potential	Access to distinctive and superior capabilities and resources
Performance	Superiority in operations and the implementation of strategy
Power	Accumulation and effective use of organizational mass

As indicated in Figure 1.1, two of these sources—power and position—focus directly on market relationships, while two—potential and performance—address distinctive internal organizational competencies. The fifth source—pace—applies equally to the internal and external sides of an organization.

Although independent as concepts, the five Ps are highly interdependent in their contributions to competitive advantage. We use the learning curve (Adler and Clark 1991; Abernathy and Wayne 1974; Henderson 1968), which is an important early concept in the field of strategy, to help us make this point.

Early entry (pace strategy) makes it possible for a competitor to move down the learning curve with time and experience, thereby lowering costs (performance strategy). Having entered early in the market, a competitor is also better able to pick from the limited talent and other resources that might be available in the market. As a result, that organization should be better able to build inimitable capabilities (potential strategy) more than might be possible for later entrants. Building on such advantages, a competitor can then expand market shares and thereby gain further advantages such as increased economies of scale (performance and power) and market clout (power). Efficiency gains can also enable a competitor to refine its position in the market, perhaps to become a low-cost provider (positioning). Alternatively, such efficiencies can lower the costs of achieving a differentiated position based on quality (positioning). Early movers might also be better able to build up consumer loyalties (positioning) and introduce switching costs (power). The relatively larger size attained by an early mover can also give that organization greater power in negotiating with both buyers and sellers in the market (power) and enable it to build up entry barriers to ward off potential entrants (power).

Clearly, strategy is a complex interweaving of ideas targeted on competitive advantage. A company can emphasize one particular source over another, considering it to be the best way by which to gain advantage, given the structures of its markets and the behaviors of and advantages available to rivals. An academic medical center might embark on an intensive positioning campaign, seeking to strengthen its identity as the high-quality provider in the marketplace. The Mayo Clinic and many other similarly prestigious referral centers, for example, have used their position as quality providers to great advantage over the years. Anticipating that local rivals might attempt to grow through mergers and acquisitions and thereby erode their distinctive positions, many of these centers have opted to preempt such moves by engaging in aggressive power strategies. The two big teaching centers in Cleveland—The Cleveland Clinic and University Hospitals Health System—are excellent examples of major institutions that pursued such a strategy. They both moved rapidly in the 1990s to gobble up the smaller community hospitals in and around Cleveland, converting the market into a near duopoly (the two split around 60 percent of the market), which is highly unusual for a market the size of Cleveland, whose population exceeds 2.25 million.

The sources of competitive advantage might also be pursued in a sequential order. A competitor might conclude that it must first establish unassailable power in its market before it seriously attempts to work on performance or to refine consumer positions. This strategy can actually be seen in the hospital sector as it transitioned from the 1990s into the 2000s. In the 1990s, many hospitals moved quickly to build up local market power through acquisitions, mergers, and partnerships. This consumed most of the available strategic energy in the hospital sector at that time. Now that many systems have formed and have achieved strong local positions of power, they appear today to be shifting their focus slightly away from power and into giving high priority to positioning strategies and to improving performance overall.

CONCLUSION

In this chapter, we define competitive strategy in terms of means (the sources of advantage) and an end (the attainment of competitive advantage). The current literature seems to be reaching a consensus on the end of strategy, but it is more ambivalent, unfortunately, about how competitive advantage should be attained.

We take an inclusive perspective regarding sources. Our view is that any source is appropriate so long as it contributes or, at least, potentially contributes to advantage and, as qualified earlier, is legal and ethical. Accordingly, we include as means not just positioning (which Porter emphasizes) and resources and capabilities (for which resource-based-view scholars advocate) but all legitimate sources of advantage. Therefore, we added to positioning and potential (our term for distinctive resources and capabilities) other sources, including power (building mass for advantage), pace (action orientation), and performance (implementation and control). All of these can provide the means by which an organization gains and sustains its advantage over its rivals.

Advantage is a relative concept, at least as applied to strategy pursued within a market context. It expresses gains made by one organization relative to those of its rivals. Certainly, organizations pursue other types of strategy that are not relative and that are more goal oriented. A hospital, for example, can have a strategy for how it plans to cope with cuts in Medicare funding, which obviously does not contrast one competitor with another. That same hospital can have a strategy for how it will handle investments in information technology. Such strategies, however, only evolve into competitive strategy when organizations view them as ways by which to gain advantage over rivals; in this sense, competitive strategy is relative. The relative framing of competitive strategy thus places the concept squarely in the context of market combat. In the beginning of this chapter, we note that strategy rose as a priority for healthcare organizations in direct correlation with the dramatic increases in the intensity of competitive skirmishing that occurred, especially in the 1990s. Put another way, competitive strategy became important when competitors began to focus on market power as a means by which to draw business away from rivals and, more generally, as a way to protect themselves against counter rival threats.

Our conceptualization of advantage in terms of the five Ps sets up much of the remaining focus of this book. We address the five Ps specifically in Chapters 5 through 9. To the extent that organizational structures are important for building or at least sustaining advantage, we consider competitive advantage in Chapter 10 as well.

REFERENCES

Abernathy, W. J., and K. Wayne. 1974. "Limits of the Learning Curve." *Harvard Business Review* 52 (5): 109–19.

Adler, P., and K. B. Clark. 1991. "Beyond the Learning Curve: A Sketch of the Learning Process." *Management Science* 37 (3): 267–81.

The Advisory Board. 1993. *The Grand Alliance*. Washington, DC: The Advisory Board.

American Hospital Association. 1990. *Section for Health Care Systems. Renewing the U.S. Health Care System*. Washington, DC: The Office of Constituency Sections.

———. 1992. *Overview: AHA's National Reform Strategy*. Chicago: American Hospital Association.

Barney, J. 1991. "Firm Resources and Sustained Competitive Advantage." *Journal of Management* 17 (1): 99–120.

Bodenheimer, T., and K. Sullivan. 1998. "How Large Employers Are Shaping the Health Care Marketplace." *New England Journal of Medicine* 338 (14): 1003–07 and 338 (15): 1084–87.

Bourgeois, L., I. Duhaime, and J. Stimpert. 1999. *Strategic Management: Concepts for Managers*, 2nd ed. Fort Worth, TX: Dryden Press.

Bracker, A. 1980. "The Historical Development of the Strategic Management Concept." *Academy of Management Review* 5 (2): 219–24.

Catholic Health Association. 1992. *Setting Relationships Right: A Working Proposal for Systemic Healthcare Reform*. St. Louis, MO: Catholic Health Association.

Chandler, A. 1977. *The Visible Hand: The Managerial Revolution in America*. Cambridge, MA: MIT Press.

Clausewitz, K. V. 2000. "Branches of the Art of War." In *The Book of War*, edited by C. Carr, 330, 390. New York: Modern Library.

Coase, R. H. 1937. "The Nature of the Firm." *Economica* 4: 386–405.

Conrad, D. A., and S. M. Shortell. 1996. "Integrated Health Services: Promises and Performance." *Frontiers of Health Services Management* 13 (1): 3–40.

D'Aveni, R. A. 1994. *Hypercompetition: Managing the Dynamics of Strategic Maneuvering*. New York: The Free Press.

Eisenhardt, K. M., and J. A. Martin. 2000. "Dynamic Capabilities: What Are They?" *Strategic Management Journal* 21 (10/11): 1105–21.

Fahey, L., and H. Christensen. 1986. "Evaluating the Research on Strategy Content." *Journal of Management* 12 (2): 167–84.

Foss, N. J. 1999. "Research in the Strategic Theory of the Firm: 'Isolationism' and 'Integrationism'." *Journal of Management Studies* 36 (6): 725–55.

Ghemawat, P. 2000. *Strategy and the Business Landscape: Core Concepts.* Upper Saddle River, NJ: Prentice Hall.

Ginter, P. M., L. E. Swayne, and W. J. Duncan. 2002. *Strategic Management of Health Care Organizations*, 4th ed. Cambridge, MA: Blackwell.

Gluck, F. W., S. P. Kaufman, and W. A. Steven. 1980. "Strategic Management for Competitive Advantage." *Harvard Business Review* 58 (5): 154–61.

Grant, R. M. 1991. "Resource-Based Theory of Competitive Advantage: Implications for Strategy Formulation." *California Management Review* 33 (3): 114–36.

Henderson, B. D. 1968. "Preface." In *Perspectives on Experience.* Boston: Boston Consulting Group.

Huff, A., and R. Reger. 1987. "Review of Strategic Process Research." *Journal of Management* 13 (2): 211–36.

Leontiades, M. 1980. *Strategies for Diversification and Change.* Boston: Little Brown and Company.

Luke, R. D., J. W. Begun, and S. L. Walston. 2000. "Strategy in Health Care Organizations and Markets." In *Health Care Management: Organizational Design and Behavior*, edited by S. Shortell and A. Kaluzny. New York: Delmar Publishers Inc.

McCraw, T. K., ed. 1998. *Creating Modern Capitalism: How Entrepreneurs, Companies, and Countries Triumphed in Three Industrial Revolutions.* Cambridge, MA: Harvard University Press.

McKiernan, P. 1997. "Strategy Past: Strategy Futures." *Long Range Planning* 30 (5): 790–98.

Merriam-Webster's Collegiate Dictionary. 2002. [Online information; retrieved 1/03.] http://www.m-w.com/cgi-bin/dictionary.

Miller, C. C., and L. B. Cardinal. 1994. "Strategic Planning and Firm Performance: A Synthesis of More Than Two Decades of Research." *Academy of Management Journal* 36 (7): 1649–65.

Mintzberg, H. 1994. *The Rise and Fall of Strategic Planning: Reconceiving Roles for Planning, Plans, Planners.* New York: The Free Press.

Montgomery, C., and M. Porter, eds. 1991. *Strategy: Seeking and Securing Competitive Advantage.* The Harvard Business Review Book Series. Boston: Harvard Business School Press.

Penrose, E. T. 1959. *The Theory of the Growth of the Firm.* Oxford, England: Basil Blackwell.

Porter, M. E. 1980. *Competitive Strategy.* New York: The Free Press.

————. 1985. *Competitive Advantage: Creating and Sustaining Superior Performance.* New York: The Free Press.

————. 1996. "What Is Strategy?" *Harvard Business Review* 74 (6): 61-78.

Powell, W. W. 1990. "Neither Market nor Hierarchy: Network Forms of Organization." In *Research in Organizational Behavior,* edited by B. M. Straw and L. L. Cummings, 295–336. Greenwich, CT: JAI Press.

Prahalad, C. K., and G. Hamel. 1994. "Strategy as a Field of Study: Why Search for a New Paradigm?" *Strategic Management Journal* 15 (1): 5–16.

Schendel, D., and C. Hoffer Schendel. 1979. *Strategic Management: A New View of Business Policy and Planning.* Boston: Little Brown and Company.

Scherer, F. M., and D. Ross. 1990. *Industrial Market Structure and Economic Performance.* Boston: Houghton Mifflin.

Schumpeter, J. A. 1942. *Capitalism, Socialism, and Democracy.* New York: Harper.

Wordsmyth: The Educational Dictionary-Thesaurus. 2002. [Online information; retrieved 1/03.] http://www.wordsmyth.net.

Chapter 2

Strategy Analysis Framework

He who knows the enemy and himself will never in a hundred battles be at risk; He who does not know the enemy but knows himself will sometimes win and sometimes lose; He who knows neither the enemy nor himself will be at risk in every battle.

—Sun-Tzu (Carr 2000, 80–81)

SUN TZU'S ASSERTION notwithstanding, systematic analyses of healthcare environments might not ensure wins in a "hundred [competitive] battles," but they should keep a healthcare organization from succumbing to the intense competitive pressures present in many markets today. The purpose of this chapter is to build the conceptual framework needed to conduct such an analysis.

Building on the discussion initiated in Chapter 1, we present the two perspectives that are currently making important contributions to strategy analysis: *market structure view* and *resource-based view*. From these views, essential concepts emerge that should be incorporated in any systematic analysis of strategy, including market structure, competitor conduct, distinctiveness, sustainability, and the value chain. We bring these concepts together into a general framework for the analysis of strategy.

This chapter highlights the need to look both inside and outside of organizations to evaluate the factors that will most likely affect the success with which strategy is formulated and implemented. In essence, we follow the admonitions of Sun Tzu: we need to know the enemy and ourselves.

FRAMING STRATEGY ANALYSIS

Prior to the 1980s, the field of strategy tended to emphasize decision-making processes more than the analysis of strategy. Mintzberg (1990)

29

associated this procedural focus with two major schools of thought on strategy formulation: design and planning. The design school concentrated on organizational processes—that is, how organizations should structure their internal processes to make strategic decisions. The planning school dealt with the many steps involved in formulating and implementing strategic plans. The design school, therefore, focused on conceptual frameworks and broad outlines, while the planning school revolved around the minutia and formality of planning.

Significantly, the two schools of thought provided few analytical prescriptions for how environments, markets, and competitors should be evaluated and related to strategic choice. As shown in Figure 2.1, both schools relegated analysis to a kind of black box, the contents of which were assumed to be understood and needed little explication. Unfortunately, the field simply had inadequate conceptual and analytical tools to assess either internal or external environments, which is the likely reason process superseded analysis in the two schools.

The field, however, has made considerable progress over the past two decades in opening up the black box of strategy analysis. Ironically, this progress is largely attributable to the work of the same two camps that butted heads over the sources of competitive advantage (see Chapter 1): the Porter camp or the market structure view (see Strategy Note 2.1) and the resource-based view proponents. Together, these two camps provide many analytical tools that are needed to evaluate, from a strategic perspective, the internal and external environments of organizations.

STRATEGY NOTE 2.1. THE PORTER PERSPECTIVE MISLABELED

Mintzberg tagged the contributions of Porter and others as the "positioning school." The reason for this label is Porter's insistence on defining strategy in terms of positioning, which captures only one of a variety of sources of competitive advantage. In reality, Porter's primary and most significant contribution is that he brought concepts and tools of industrial organization economics to the field of strategy, which greatly enhanced the analytical power of the strategy analyst. In this book, therefore, we refer to this perspective as the market structure view.

Figure 2.1. The Black Box of the Design and Planning Schools of Thought

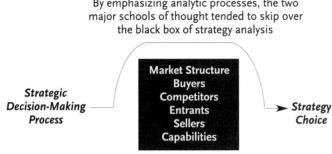

In Figure 2.2, we fit the two perspectives within that classic framework known by the acronym *SWOT* [strengths, weaknesses, opportunities, and threats] (Henderson 1979; Andrews 1971). The resource-based view focuses on internal strengths and weaknesses, while the market structure view centers around external threats and opportunities. Note that swot should be viewed as a general conceptualization, not as a formula or formal tool per se. Despite its widely recognized face validity, swot has its limitations (Hill and Westbrook 1997). For further discussion of swot, see Strategy Tool A at the end of this chapter.

Market Structure View

Markets are possibly the most immediate and obvious factor to consider in conducting a strategy analysis. Market structures and the patterns of competitor behavior are the essential features of markets that strategists need to understand. The theoretical underpinnings for the study of market structure come from the field of *industrial organization* (io) economics, which came into being when economists began to diverge from the orthodox assumptions associated with perfectly competitive markets. The latter markets are characterized by large numbers of competitors, none of which possess sufficient power to affect prices or the behaviors of competitors. Once the assumption of small numbers was relaxed, competitors could no longer be assumed to be without market power. So the models of competition sought to understand how competitors might use market power to affect prices and the behaviors of rivals (Coase 1937; Schumpeter 1942; Penrose 1959). Because such models deal with the

Figure 2.2. SWOT and the Two Major Perspectives on Strategy

Opportunities	Threats	*Market Structure View (External)*
Strengths	Weaknesses	*Resource-Based View (Internal)*

exercise of market power, they also provide an important foundation for understanding competition and strategy.

Foundations of the Industrial Organization Economics Model

Building on the early theorizing, Mason (1939) and others (Clark 1940; Bain 1959; Clark 1961) postulated the causal sequence of determinants that could influence the conduct of competitors as collectives. As presented in Figure 2.3, the resulting model identifies environmental and market structures as the primary drivers of competitor conduct, and these three together—environmental and market structures and competitor conduct—as the determinants of market outcomes or performance.

Structure, the central concept in the model, refers to a wide variety of market characteristics that influence the behaviors of competitors. Three of these characteristics are among the most prominent: *market concentration* (number and size distribution of organizations), *entry barriers*, and the degree of *product differentiation* (Bain and Qualls 1987). (Market structure is discussed in greater detail in Chapter 4. For some definitions of key concepts, see Strategy Note 2.2.)

Extensive research (Chandler 1962; Rumelt 1974) and coherent and comprehensive scholarly expositions (Scherer and Ross 1990) followed the

Figure 2.3. Industrial Organization Economics Model

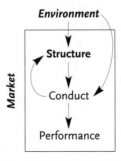

STRATEGY NOTE 2.2. DEFINITIONS

Environment: External factors (not otherwise included in market structure) that play or are likely to play an important role in influencing the structures of markets, conduct of rivals, and strategies of individual firms.

Market: An arena in which one or more sellers of given products and their close substitutes exchange with and compete for the patronage of a group of buyers. Markets are typically delimited in geographic (e.g., metropolitan areas) or product terms (e.g., general acute medical/surgical care) or both.

Market Structure: The organizational features of a market that condition or influence the conduct and strategies of organizations.

Conduct: The collective* actions that organizations take within markets in pursuit of competitive advantage.

* For our purposes, both conduct and strategy refer to the strategic behaviors of competitors. The difference is that conduct refers to the collective and strategy applies to individual competitors.

---

early conceptualizations of market structure and conduct. As a result, IO became the primary branch through which the concepts and theories of economics are now applied to the study of markets.

Endogeneity in the Model

Understand that the causal sequence linking structure and conduct is not unidirectional. As shown in Figure 2.3, market structure is itself endogenous—that is, it affects and is influenced by market conduct (Bain and Qualls 1987). This means that although the many strategic decisions competitors make (to engage in merger and acquisition activities, for example) may be conditioned by the structures of their markets, those same strategic maneuvers can and often do forge changes in the structures themselves.

The *endogeneity of market structure* actually played itself out in the 1990s when healthcare markets underwent significant restructuring. Facing increasing concentration in buyer markets (change in structure), hospitals reacted by engaging in merger and acquisition behaviors (collectively, a change in market conduct), a consequence of which was dramatically increased levels of concentration of their markets (an endogenous impact on market structure). The drivers, responses, and counter responses of the hospitals together reveal the bidirectional relationship (endogeneity) that exists between individual and collective competitor decisions and market structures.

Interestingly, a similar and possibly more powerful strategy-structure interaction occurred in the supply-distribution channel. Anticipating consolidation among both providers and managed care organizations (a change in the buyer structure), healthcare distributors aggressively engaged in mergers and acquisitions (a change in conduct) to gain positions of power that could help them offset the growing power of their buyers and their immediate rivals. Consequently, distributor markets consolidated (a change in structure) still further, the result of which is that a handful of major suppliers now dominate healthcare distribution nationwide.

Market Structure and Strategy

The concepts and tools of IO were not widely used in strategy analysis until after Porter published his book on competitive strategy in 1980. The reason is that IO is concerned mostly with evaluating the performance of markets and using such evaluations to inform public policy of the role government should play in ensuring that resources are allocated efficiently and prices are set competitively. A *policy question* addressed from an IO perspective, for example, might be "How do oligopolistic market structures under conditions of, say, high product differentiation, affect price competition?" A related policy question might be "What interventions are needed to ensure that the markets produce real price competition and the most efficient utilization of resources?" IO would not then go further to ask, "What should a specific organization do to survive under such market conditions?" That question, which would not be the focus of IO or policy, falls directly within the domain of strategy analysis.

Since publication of Porter's book, the structural perspective has dominated analytic thinking in the field (a point made by Mintzberg in his 1990 and 1998 works). Porter's book produced a conceptual windfall for both students and practitioners of strategy, filling in one of the most critical gaps in the analytic frame (and in the black box discussed earlier): the study of the interrelationships among markets, competitors, and strategy. Porter's "five forces" model (see Figure 2.4) captures diagrammatically the practical extension of IO to organizational strategy. The model shifts the focus to individual organizations and away from collectives, and it expands the number and variety of structural factors one might need to consider in strategy analysis. These factors include threats (which come in a wide

Figure 2.4. Porter's Five Forces Framework

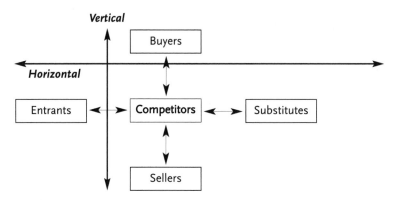

Source: Adapted with the permission of The Free Press, a Division of Simon & Schuster Adult Publishing Group, from COMPETITIVE STRATEGY: Techniques for Analyzing Industries and Competitors by Michael E. Porter. Copyright © 1980, 1998 by The Free Press.

variety of forms detailed in Chapter 4), not just from competitors and buyers but from sellers, substitutes, and potential entrants as well.

The five forces are arrayed in Figure 2.4 both vertically (between buyers, competitors, and sellers) and horizontally (between entrants, competitors, and substitutes). The horizontal structure represents existing and potential rivals, and the vertical structure signifies threats inherent in buyer-seller relationships. Obviously, threats from one's immediate competitors are the most important of the five. Typically, rivals are in the best position to undermine any market advantages a given organization might have gained. Here is where the effects of conventional IO structures—market concentration, entry barriers, and product differentiation—come directly into view.

Within each of the five forces, Porter examined a number of specific structural factors that could shape the intensity of rivalry and the specifics of an organization's strategic choice. These factors include, for example, the presence (or absence) of high fixed costs, economies of scale, over (or under) capacity, high (or low) rates of market growth, switching costs, and so forth. All such factors are elements of market structure and should be incorporated into the analysis of strategy.

No one structural driver should be overemphasized in strategy analysis without good reason. To do so would be to risk underspecifying the determinants of competitive advantage. The well-known Boston Consulting Group (BCG) Grid (Stern and Stalk 1998), for example, does just this; it gives undue emphasis to a single structural indicator—market growth. (The second measure used in the BCG model—market share—is actually an indicator of the strategic position of the individual business units owned by multibusiness organizations, and it is not a measure of market structure per se.) Certainly, market growth is important and should be considered in any thorough analysis of strategy; however, most markets are just too complex for any one indicator to be evaluated in isolation. Subsequent models developed to replace the BCG Grid have incorporated a much wider array of factors into the analysis of strategic choice, including the GE Business Screen (Majluf and Hax 1983). (The BCG Grid and GE Business Screen are discussed further in Chapter 7.) One of Porter's important contributions, therefore, was that he increased the complexity of analysis by expanding the number of market structural factors to consider when analyzing strategy.

Resource-Based View

The second major perspective that has contributed tools to the analysis of strategy is the resource-based view. The central idea underlying this perspective is that organizations gain competitive advantage by successfully assembling and utilizing valuable and distinctive resources and capabilities. Both are important: resources are the tangible elements within organizations—manpower, plant, equipment, location, to name a few; capabilities are the intangibles—talent, skills, management systems, coordinating mechanisms, experience, organizational knowledge, and other distinguishing organizational abilities. Because they are so basic to organizations, both resources and capabilities are easily overlooked as possible sources of advantage. (To avoid the unnecessary replication of terms, we will henceforth use the term "resources" when referring to the combination of resources and capabilities.)

Capabilities are especially easy to overlook because they are often very complex, subtle, and poorly understood. Most hospitals in a market, for example, will have reasonably competent management staffs, but one might have a particularly well integrated management team that is, as a result, especially adept at coordination, group decision making, and responding rapidly to changes in the market. Such distinctiveness in capabilities may not be easy to recognize or attribute to gains in competitive advantage. A unique feature of capabilities is that they are often the product of organizational learning, although they can be acquired as well. Thus, they often evolve over time and, as a result, are commonly taken for granted.

An organization's capabilities can be either deep or shallow, a difference that is important to understand in their evaluation. Capabilities are shallow when they are not tied to specific products, services, markets, or customer bases. Capabilities are deep when they have more specific and targeted applications. Therefore, *deep capabilities* might provide organizations with immediate advantages in particular areas, while *shallow capabilities* might enable organizations to succeed in a variety of areas as well as over time in the face of changing market circumstances. Depending on an organization's purpose, deep capabilities can produce long-run benefits as well, such as might be achieved in building depth in a selected clinical area that is then used to establish a strong position of quality in the marketplace. Unfortunately, the strategic potential of resources and capabilities is inadequately understood or appreciated by most organizations engaged in strategy analyses.

Distinctiveness

The suggestion that resources might produce market advantages for an organization can be traced very far back to a theory first propounded by the economist David Ricardo (1817). He explained that advantages accrue to those organizations that gain access to superior resources, if those resources are not evenly distributed among competitors because of imperfections in factor or input markets. The central idea in Ricardo's theory, as well as in the resource-based view, is that access to specific resources needs to be limited or *distinctive* if those resources are to have any impact on competition (see Strategy Note 2.3).

In more recent times, scholars have suggested a number of characteristics that are required for resources to be strategic (Collis and Montgomery 1995; Grant 1998; Barney 1996). These characteristics fall into two general categories: (1) *strategic importance* and (2) *sustainability*. A resource, even if highly important strategically, provides little advantage if it can be duplicated easily by rivals. Rarity, uniqueness, the presence of barriers to access (e.g., patents), and so forth enhance sustainability. On the other hand, a sustainable capability that makes no discernable contribution to strategy will produce little advantage.

The strategic importance of resources is derived in two ways. First, resources, especially those that are visible to and highly valued by consumers, make *direct contributions* to competitive advantage. Healthcare consumers often place a high value on such features as exceptional clinical manpower, modern facilities, good parking, and favorable locations. Second, resources

STRATEGY NOTE 2.3. MONOPOLY POWER OR SUPERIOR RESOURCES?

Advantage under the Ricardian reasoning is not grounded in the buildup of monopoly power as might be derived from external market strategies, such as product positioning, or the buildup of market shares and dominance (which, of course, is the emphasis of the market structure view). Rather, advantage derives from what Ricardo referred to as *economic "rents"*—premiums earned on resources over their opportunity costs or above what might be expected given market conditions.

The resource-based-view proponents, having adopted the Ricardian perspective, often argue against the external sources of market power as the basis for competitive advantage. Peteraf (1993, 180–81), for example, argued that superior resources are what count, not market dominance:

> The high returns of efficient firms cannot be attributed to an artificial restriction of output or to market power…that is the key is that the superior resources remain limited in supply. Thus efficient firms can sustain this type of competitive advantage only if their resources cannot be expanded freely or imitated by other firms.

A more balanced view, we suggest, is that both are important; superior resources, efficiencies, and profitability are integrally linked to an organization's ability to take those market actions needed to build market power and vice versa. Grant (1998, 183) acknowledged this relationship between rents and market power, although, oddly, he used this relationship to make the case for the resource-based view over the market structural view:

> …business strategy should be viewed less as a quest for monopoly rents (the returns to market power) and more as a quest for Ricardian rents (the returns to the resources which confer competitive advantage over and above the real costs of those resources)…. We can go further. A closer look at

market power and the monopoly rent it offers suggests that it too has its basis in the resources of firms. The fundamental prerequisite for market power is the presence of barriers to entry. Barriers to entry are based upon scale economies, patents, experience advantages, brand reputation, or some other resource which incumbent firms possess but which entrants can acquire only slowly or at disproportionate expense.

Grant is saying that even if monopoly power produces advantage (which it obviously does), that power is nevertheless grounded in the possession by the dominating organization of distinctive resources and capabilities, which potential entrants might have difficulty duplicating.

The linkage between monopoly power and superior resources is helpful, but the exclusionary argument favoring internal over external positions is not. Both are important and are mutually reinforcing. Gains in monopoly power are often dependent on much more than superior resources. Grant's point that market share depends on efficiencies, for example, is only partially correct. Market share is also tied to a variety of internal and external strategic actions, including successful positioning, pursuit of mergers and acquisitions, aggressive decisions to enter markets early, and so forth. The representatives of the two perspectives should now set aside their self-interested and defensive arguments and forge an integration of ideas that enlightens us on how organizations go about building competitive advantage.

that are less visible or even entirely invisible to or not understood by the consuming public can make *indirect contributions* to competitive advantage. They do this by enhancing other sources of competitive advantage. For example, a well-developed capability to adapt to changing market or environmental change might not be visible to outsiders but can have a major impact on the timing of an organization's moves in the market or the success with which its positioning strategies are introduced. The same would be true for resources such as a powerful and effective information system; deep pockets that can fuel an aggressive strategic agenda; or, for a drug company, a patent on a highly popular prescription drug. In competition with Kmart, for example, Wal-Mart invested heavily in building efficient operations and distribution systems, with an emphasis on information technologies. Little immediate advantage might have been visible in the market except, perhaps, in Wal-Mart's ability to offer slightly lower prices. A major (often invisible) advantage for Wal-Mart, however, is its ability to survive market downturns, which is a result of having established more efficient internal systems of control and distribution.

In any case, resources must affect advantage, not just be superior. Put another way, internal resources do little good if, in effect, they are bottled up inside an organization, dormant, or ineffectually applied to strategy.

Expanding the Essential Conditions

Building on the work of Barney (1997), Bourgeois, Duhaime, and Stimpert (1999) expanded the conditions of importance and sustainability as follows:

1. Strategic importance: valuable, it actually produces advantage.
2. Sustainability: rare, difficult to imitate, and difficult to substitute.
3. Duration: time over which the advantage is sustainable.

As can be seen, Bourgeois, Duhaime, and Stimpert added a time dimension to the analysis, suggesting that imitating a rival's sources of advantage may not be feasible in the short term but may be possible over the long haul. Figure 2.5 is our adaptation of their analysis of the criteria combined with time. In the figure, the two major dimensions are arrayed in a hierarchical order, building inclusively from strategic importance, as the most basic requirement for advantage, to sustainable (not duplicable) over the long term, the highest-level requirement for advantage.

If an organization's resources meet none of these characteristics, then, as suggested in the figure, no advantage will be produced. A resource that is valuable and possibly rare, but inimitable or substitutable even in the short term, will produce only a transitory competitive advantage. A competitive but not necessarily sustainable advantage might be achieved if that advantage can be sustained in the short term, but not over time. Ultimately, a truly sustainable advantage would result only when a distinctive and strategically important resource cannot be imitated or substituted even in the long run.

Although the concepts of importance and sustainability are important from a resource-based perspective, they should not be restricted to the

Figure 2.5. Hierarchy of Advantages Attributable to Organizational Resources and Capabilities

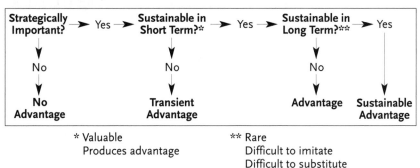

Source: Concept from Bourgeois, L., Il. Duhaime, and J. Stimpert. 1999. *Strategic Management: Concepts for Managers*, 2nd ed. Fort Worth, TX: Dryden Press.

analysis of resources and capabilities alone. Indeed, they apply to all sources of advantage, whether internally or externally based. They apply, for example, to positioning. Even if a competitor were to achieve a low-cost position in the marketplace, that position would produce little advantage if rivals can easily replicate it. Also, they apply to power strategies. If a competitor gains advantage by building up organizational scale and consequent market power, but its most immediate rival is able to counter this by merging with remaining rivals, that advantage can very possibly be neutralized. This does not mean that such a move is not warranted, but that it might not be sustainable over time. Clearly, strategy analysts must apply the above conditions (and others, as appropriate) when assessing any of the sources of advantage.

Activities and the Value Chain

Ironically, Porter (1985), who is most prominently associated with the market structure perspective, has also contributed to the analysis of internal organizational factors. Specifically, he argued that for organizations to carve out distinctive cost and differentiation positions (external advantages), they must carefully assess and integrate the various activities they perform in producing goods and services.

Activities represent a somewhat different conceptualization than do resources and capabilities. They comprise the many functions that organizations perform in the conduct of business, including marketing, producing, distributing, acquiring, financing, and so forth. Ghemawat (2001, 117) referred to activities as the "flows" or strategic tasks that competitors perform in the pursuit of advantage (and he characterized resources and capabilities as the "stocks" that facilitate those flows and delimit their market potential). Porter introduced the concept of a *value chain* to highlight all such activities within organizations that can conceivably affect costs and success in achieving distinctiveness in the market. Competitors are expected to scrutinize each of the activities within their value chains and to seek ways to improve the congruence, complementariness, or fit among their various activities, including their joint effects on competitive advantage.

Porter (1996) used the remarkable success of Southwest Airlines to illustrate how better management (better fit, consistency, synergy) of the activities within an organization's value chain translates into successful positioning. (Remember, Porter restricts strategy to positioning.) Rather than seek mergers and acquisitions to compete directly against other airlines, as many major airlines had done, Southwest carefully manipulated its product and management strategies to help it succeed in the often overlooked shorter-route niche. To do this, Southwest limited the costly passenger-support activities that are common to most airlines. Few amenities were provided: no connections to other airlines were arranged; no baggage transfers were allowed; no seats were assigned as passengers picked their seats on a first-come, first-serve basis; on-time departures were stressed; and so forth. These activity adjustments in how Southwest went about its business enabled the airline to streamline many of its service-heavy activities and, amazingly, to lower ticket prices on typically costly low-volume routes. Southwest thus combined the restructuring of internal management activities with an attempt to achieve a distinctive position as a low-cost competitor.

The focus on activities and value chains is very useful because it reemphasizes the significant extent to which external sources of advantage are dependent not only on the way products are presented in the market (externally), but also on the many important tasks organizations perform on a daily basis (internally). This idea is especially germane to the healthcare industry, given the high levels of intimacy and simultaneity that exist between providers and patients during the delivery of services. It is easy to see how the internal workings of provider systems might affect the attitudes of patients and others who view those internal workings first hand. Thus, it is reasonable to expect that analyses of the value chains of healthcare organizations will prove particularly beneficial in the organizations' attempts to enhance their market positions as well as to gain other competitive advantages. Porter stressed the relationship between the management of activities and positioning, but better management of such activities obviously can enhance many other sources of advantage as well (see the Wal-Mart example above), even if positioning per se is not affected directly.

Also, the value chain concept can be applied to all levels and combinations of organizations, including individual departments, business units, corporations, vertical partners, and even the vast array of interrelated and often loosely interconnected delivery entities that comprise local or regional healthcare delivery systems. Given their importance to the analysis of strategy, we revisit these ideas in Chapter 6.

A SUMMARY FRAMEWORK FOR STRATEGY ANALYSIS

Now, let us integrate the two perspectives—resource based and market structure—into a framework for the analysis of strategy. We begin by introducing a decision framework that incorporates the three internal elements identified thus far—resources, capabilities, and activities.

Strategy-Choice Sequence

Ghemawat (2001, 111–35) provided a helpful starting point for this integration by linking the resource-based and activities approaches together as essential components of strategic decision making. We have modified Ghemawat's logic to fit the framework directly to our purposes; this approach is illustrated in Figure 2.6. (This framework does not include analyses of external environments, which we incorporate into our final framework.)

In Figure 2.6, resource commitments is placed after decisions about strategy; Ghemawat, on the other hand, placed this item sequentially before activities analysis. His argument was that resource commitments are necessary for activities to move forward, which of course is logical. We are interested, however, in framing these as a sequence of strategic decisions. In this case, the analysis of all internal factors (activities, resources, and capabilities) form a basis on which strategic ideas are adopted, and based on those ideas, resources are committed. Remember, strategy is made up of concepts and ideas that guide organizations in their pursuit of competitive advantage. Once adopted, those ideas should provide organizations with the direction needed to commit resources. A feedback loop has been included in the framework, noting that new funding and resource commitments affect the three internal elements (resources, capabilities, and activities).

Figure 2.6. A Dynamic View of the Resource-Based Perspective

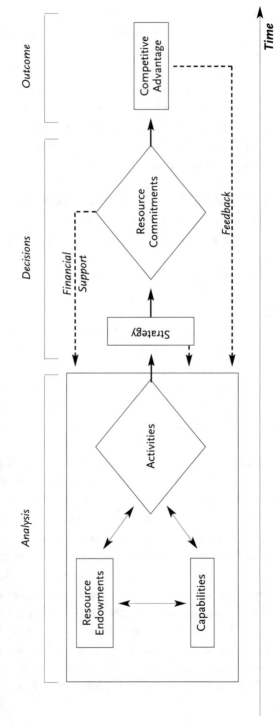

Source: Concepts from Ghemawat, P. 2001. *Strategy and the Business Landscape: Core Concepts,* 111–35. Upper Saddle River, NJ: Prentice-Hall.

Constructing the Framework

The strategy analysis process is presented in Figure 2.7. We bring together the two major perspectives—market structure and resource-based views—in configuring a comprehensive analytic frame for examining the impact of internal and external factors on strategy. The market structure view model is on the right of the figure, and the resource-based view model (using the revised Ghemawat version as presented in Figure 2.6) is on the left. As shown, the external analysis feeds into the internal analysis; together, these lead to strategic decisions, commitments of resources, and, hopefully, competitive advantage.

Some organizations will find more value in emphasizing one environment over another (internal versus external). Assessments of internal environments might be essential for a hospital system that enjoys a near monopoly in a market; such is the case for the Carilion Health System in Roanoke, Virginia, which maintains about a 75 percent market share in the local urban area. Having well-established market positions, such systems might be expected to focus less on rivals and more on ensuring that they are able to sustain, and perhaps expand, their control over their markets. This could lead Carilion, for example, to focus on assessing its internal value chain (to better align its internal functioning with its intended market positions) or to emphasize integration for purposes of cost control. By contrast, a system located in a more contentious market environment might choose a different emphasis. Such might be the case for Texas Health Resources (THR), a 12-hospital local system located in the urban cluster of Fort Worth and Dallas. THR has a dominant position in Fort Worth, with just over 40 percent of the acute care market, but it is in third position in the nearby, larger, and more competitive Dallas market. Given the uncertainties inherent in the latter market, THR might be expected to emphasize external factors (such as further acquisitions or mergers in Dallas) to achieve greater parity with rivals there. In Fort Worth, on the other hand, THR might instead focus on those strategies (with a possible emphasis on internal elements) that help to maintain its strength in that market.

Many hospitals gave very high priority to external factors in the heady days of the 1990s. They did this to countervail threats from managed care companies, hospital rivals, and physician organizations. Having succeeded in building up market power and facing less competitor threats (possibly temporarily) in their market environments, many of those same competitors today are shifting their attention to internal sources of competitive advantage, improving efficiencies, obtaining more sophisticated information

Figure 2.7. Strategy Analysis Framework

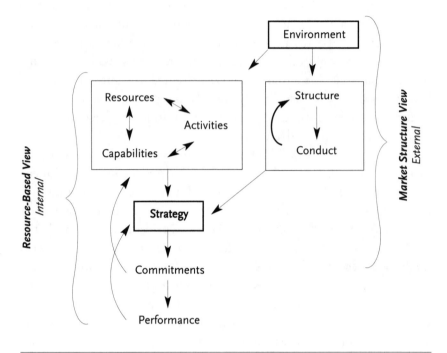

systems, consolidating among owned facilities, and so forth. Each important shift that occurs in the broader and market environments is likely to be accompanied by corresponding reordering of the relative weights assigned to internal versus external factors. Strategy analysts thus must be adaptive and thoughtful in pursuing strategy, which is all the more important in today's rapidly and ever-changing environment. (For a discussion of scenario analysis as a method for assessing trends in the external environment, see Strategy Tool B at the end of this chapter.)

CONCLUSION

In this chapter, the overall framework for conducting a thorough strategy analysis is developed. The somewhat simplistic and often overused SWOT framework still stands the test of time as a general guide in analyzing strategy. Certainly, external factors (opportunities and threats), such as the broader environment, market structure, and competitor conduct, need to be evaluated. Similarly, internal factors (strengths and weaknesses), such as resources, capabilities, and activities, need to be assessed, even if their connection to competitive advantage might not be so easily deduced.

The concepts derived from IO economics provide the essential foundation for assessing external factors. Porter's (and those who followed him) translation of those concepts and his linkage of those concepts to market strategy allow us to have a clearer understanding of how different market structures point to different approaches to market strategy. Very possibly, the most difficult aspects to analyze are the internal resources that can make such an important difference in the degree to which an organization is able to gain and sustain advantage. Scholars associated with the resource-based view have therefore made an important contribution by highlighting the characteristics of resources and capabilities that are needed to ensure advantage.

The framework in this chapter provides the backdrop for understanding the content presented in the remainder of this book. Keeping such a framework in mind is important because, unfortunately, strategy is rarely the product of a formularized or tidy analytical process. Institutional constraints, shifting market forces, and pure irrationality are the hallmarks of strategic decision making. Therefore, the analyst must surround the analytical process with as much conceptual ordering as needed to give some rationality to the vagary and capriciousness of strategic decision making.

REFERENCES

Andrews, K. R. 1971. *The Concept of Corporate Strategy*. Homewood, IL: Irwin.

Bain, J. S. 1959. Industrial Organization. New York: John Wiley.

Bain, J. S., and D. Qualls. 1987. *Industrial Organization: A Treatise*, Volume 6, Part A. Greenwich, CT: JAI Press.

Barney, J. 1991. "Firm Resources and Sustained Competitive Advantage." *Journal of Management* 17 (1): 99–120.

———. 1996. "The Resource-Based Theory of the Firm." *Organizational Science* 7 (5): 469.

———.1997. *Gaining and Sustaining Competitive Advantages*. Reading, MA: Addison-Wesley.

Bourgeois, L., I. Duhaime, and J. Stimpert. 1999. *Strategic Management: Concepts for Managers*, 2nd ed. Fort Worth, TX: Dryden Press.

Carr, C., ed. 2000. "Planning the Attack," translated from Sun Tzu. In *The Book of War*, 80–81. New York: Modern Library.

Chandler, A. D., Jr. 1962. *Strategy and Structure*. Cambridge, MA: MIT Press.

Clark, J. M. 1940. "Toward a Concept of Workable Competition." *American Economic Review* 30 (2): 241–56.

———. 1961. *Competition as a Dynamic Process*. New York: Brookings Institution.

Coase, R. H. 1937. "The Nature of the Firm." *Economica* 4: 386–405.

Collis, D., and C. Montgomery. 1995. "Competing on Resources: Strategy in the 1990s." *Harvard Business Review* 73 (4): 118–28.

Ghemawat, P. 2001. *Strategy and the Business Landscape: Core Concepts.* Upper Saddle River, NJ: Prentice-Hall.

Grant, R. 1998. "The Resource-Based Theory of Competitive Advantage: Implications for Strategy Formulation." In *The Strategy Reader*, edited by S. Segal-Horn, 179–99. Malden, MA: Blackwell.

Henderson, B. D. 1979. *On Corporate Strategy.* Cambridge, MA: Abt Books.

Hill, T., and R. Westbrook. 1997. "SWOT Analysis: It's Time for a Product Recall." *Long Range Planning* 30 (1): 46–52.

Majluf, S., and A. Hax. 1983. "The Use of the Growth-Share Matrix in Strategic Planning." *Interfaces* 13 (2): 46–60.

Mason, E. S. 1939. "Price and Production Policies of Large Scale Enterprise." *The American Economic Review* 29 (1): 61–74.

Mintzberg, H. 1990. "Strategy Formation: Schools of Thought." In *Perspectives on Strategic Management*, edited by J. W. Fredrickson, Chapter 5. New York: Harper Business.

———. 1998. *Strategy Safari: A Guided Tour Through the Wilds of Strategic Management.* New York: The Free Press.

Penrose, E. T. 1959. *The Theory of the Growth of the Firm.* Oxford, England: Basil Blackwell.

Peteraf, M. 1993. "The Cornerstones of Competitive Advantage: A Resource-Based View." *Strategic Management Journal* 14 (3): 179–91.

Porter, M. 1980. *Competitive Strategy.* New York: The Free Press.

———. 1985. *Competitive Advantage: Creating and Sustaining Superior Performance.* New York: The Free Press.

———. 1996. "What Is Strategy?" *Harvard Business Review* 74 (6): 61–78.

Ricardo, D. 1817. *On the Principles of Political Economy and Taxation.* London: John Murray.

Rumelt, R. P. 1974. *Strategy, Structure, and Economic Performance.* Boston: Harvard Business School.

Scherer, F. M., and D. Ross. 1990. *Industrial Market Structure and Economic Performance.* Boston: Houghton Mifflin.

Schumpeter, J. A. 1942. *Capitalism, Socialism, and Democracy.* New York: Harper.

Stern, C. W., and G. Stalk, eds. 1998. *Perspectives on Strategy: From the Boston Consulting Group.* New York: John Wiley & Sons.

STRATEGY TOOL A. SWOT ANALYSIS

SWOT is possibly the most commonly used analytical tool in strategy analysis because it is simple and intuitive. The purpose of a SWOT analysis is to isolate key issues that are expected to drive strategy choice.

Many strategic retreats open with some variation of a SWOT analysis. This is because SWOT provides a good way to summarize key points about organizations—specifically, their strengths (S), weaknesses (W), opportunities (O), and threats (T). This summary allows managers collectively to perceive the good, bad, and potential for their organizations. Perhaps most usefully, SWOT is a situational analysis tool that serves as an interpretive filter through which key strategic issues can readily be evaluated. SWOT often serves as a useful frame for shaping brainstorming sessions, surveys, and other information-collecting efforts.

The following describes how a SWOT analysis can be developed through a brainstorming situational analysis and then broken down into internal and external analyses that become a SWOT profile.

Brainstorming SWOT

As in any brainstorming situation, a nonthreatening environment should be created to allow free flow of information. A leader or facilitator should have control of the session, clearly charging the group to develop a meaningful SWOT analysis. Also, the leader should encourage participation and an enthusiastic, uncritical attitude from all participants. Participants should come from various parts of the organization. Those who participate in brainstorming should be encouraged to come up with many ideas and to be as creative as possible. The leader should not allow ideas to be criticized or evaluated during the brainstorming session. A record should be kept of the session either as notes or a tape recording. Also helpful is to jot down ideas on a board that can be seen by all participants. The brainstorming session should be divided into the components of SWOT.

The internal analysis consists of evaluating the strengths and weaknesses of internal organizational resources, capabilities, and activities, which exist in the following areas:

- Company culture
- Company image
- Organizational structure
- Key staff
- Access to key resources

- Position on the experience curve
- Operational efficiency
- Operational capacity
- Brand awareness
- Market share
- Financial resources
- Exclusive contracts
- External relationships
- Interorganizational/integrative structure
- IT capabilities
- Administrative processes
- Clinical control processes
- Strategic decision-making processes

The following are potential questions to pose during internal analyses.

Strengths
- What are the organization's distinctive resources and capabilities? How do they compare to those of competitors'?
- If customers were asked, what would they *see* as the organization's strengths?
- If competitors were asked, what would they *say* were the organization's strengths?

Weaknesses
- What resources and capabilities need improvement in the organization?
- What distinctive resources and capabilities do our primary competitors have that we might need to duplicate?
- What should the organization avoid doing?
- What is done now in the organization that creates problems and complaints?
- Are there system failures in the organization?
- Are there integrative failures in the organization?

Next, the external environment should be examined, with its attendant opportunities and threats. The following are areas in which opportunities and threats might exist:

- Customers/buyers
- Competitors
- Substitutes
- Potential entrants
- Suppliers
- Partners
- Physicians
- Market structure
- Market trends
- Social changes
- New technology
- Economic environment
- Political and regulatory environment

Opportunities
- What opportunities are available to the organization?
- Are there neglected market positions in which the competitors are weak?
- What are the interesting trends on which the organization might capitalize?
- Are there advantages currently enjoyed by competitors that can be eroded?
- Do any of the members of the organization's "strategic group" (see Chapter 4) do things that the organization might need to consider?

Threats
- What are the most serious obstacles/trends faced by the organization?
- Are there specific threats from buyers? Sellers? Substitutes? Entrants? Existing rivals?
- Is changing technology threatening the organization's position and/or operational efficiencies?
- Can rivals easily erode the organization's existing sources of competitive advantage?
- Does the organization lack the financial means to accomplish the needed strategic moves for the future? Does it lack the needed staff? Does it lack needed capabilities, processes, and systems?

When the analysis is completed, a SWOT profile can be generated and used as the basis for goal setting, strategy formulation, and strategy implementation. Sometimes, a completed SWOT profile is arranged as follows:

Strengths	Weaknesses	Opportunities	Threats
1.	1.	1.	1.
2.	2.	2.	2.
3.	3.	3.	3.

When formulating strategy, the interaction of the quadrants in the SWOT profile becomes important. For example, the strengths may be leveraged to pursue opportunities and to avoid threats, and managers can be alerted to weaknesses that might need to be overcome to successfully pursue opportunities. Upon completion of the SWOT analysis, make sure that the information is used to change the strategic behavior of the organization. One can do this by categorizing each point according to the following:

- Things that must be addressed immediately
- Things that can be handled now
- Things that should be researched further
- Things that should be planned for the future

Then, each item should be prioritized, action plans should be established, time frames should be established, and responsibility for follow-up should be given to individuals.

Another way to use a SWOT analysis for strategic direction is by arraying the factors and then determining a suggested strategy based on the mix of factors. Different matrixes can be constructed in which those factors most relevant to a particular strategy might be included. A degree of importance can be ascribed by listing SWOT components by their number or magnitude. The factors then can be added and a numerical score obtained for each segment.

The Use of Surveys

Some of the questions asked during a SWOT analysis can only be addressed through surveys. Surveys can be used to assemble information from customers, employees, physicians, and the general public. These would not be formal "research" surveys but intelligence-collecting exercises. Thus, they should be simple, highly targeted, and limited in the number of persons contacted (to reduce the cost and time needed to gather the information). The surveys are thus useful for generating general insights, hints, and other information. General guidelines on formulating surveys for purposes of strategy analysis include the following:

1. Ask questions in a logical sequence.
2. Frame questions without using technical terms.
3. Avoid hypothetical questions; instead, focus on the specific points.
4. Have each question require only one answer to avoid confusion.
5. Avoid words with double meanings.
6. Avoid words that are emotionally charged.
7. Give options that are exclusive, and try to include all of the possible responses when asking closed questions.
8. Place open-ended or controversial questions at the end of the survey.
9. Survey a statistically adequate number of people.

Problems with SWOT Analyses

Although many organizations frequently use SWOT analyses, their use is fraught with problems. Probably the most serious of these is the potential subjectivity of the analysis. This is highlighted by the tendency to oversimplify by categorizing environmental and internal factors into two categories. For example, an organization's culture might be a strength for one portion of the business and a weakness in another. Assessments will also be biased by the managers' perception of organizational strengths and weaknesses. Organizations with many strengths often perceive environmental changes as opportunities; similarly, those with weaknesses will see these changes as threats. Another issue with a SWOT analysis is that its use often does not lead to any clear-cut recommendations. Few organizations have only strengths and opportunities; most have a mix of all four factors. A SWOT analysis is also only a snapshot in time and does not include longitudinal estimates of the sustainability of advantages and the persistence of disadvantages. Finally, SWOT is simply too general: it offers only a starting point for analysis. To enhance this framework, one would need to draw on the available conceptual and analytical tools, especially those found within the market structure and resource-based views.

STRATEGY TOOL B. SCENARIO ANALYSIS

Scenario analysis has emerged as a useful tool for assessing intended strategies in the context of possible future developments. Traditionally, estimations of the future are based on projections of existing environmental trends. However, as with the weather, today's conditions might provide only slightly better predictions of the future than would a mere flip of a coin. Nevertheless, humans tend to view the future very much in the context of the present, as the following predictions imply:

"Who the hell wants to hear actors talk?" (H. M. Warner of Warner Brothers, speaking in 1927 when weekly cinema attendance was about 5 million a week. By the end of 1929, "talking pictures" were drawing 90 million people a week)

"A severe depression like that of 1920–1921 is outside the range of probability." (The Harvard Economic Society on November 16, 1929, when the Great Depression in the United States was just beginning)

"Atomic energy might be as good as our present day explosives, but it is unlikely to produce anything very much more dangerous." (Winston Churchill in 1939, years before the first atomic bomb was dropped, killing and injuring thousands of people)

"The bomb will never go off. I speak as an expert in explosives." (Admiral William Leahy, speaking in 1943 about the Manhattan Project, the U.S. government initiative during World War II to build an atomic bomb)

These highly capable, influential individuals appear to have relied on existing facts to make erroneous projections about the future. Frequently, devising strategies do the same. However, predicting future environmental and competitive conditions is very much an art; it is imprecise and fraught with error.

Scenario analysis allows organizations to consider multiple futures and to evaluate strategies under varying future conditions. As a result, it is very valuable for assessing future contingencies and conducting sensitivity analyses or "what if" analyses.

The assessment of alternative futures allows analysts to account for some of the uncertainties that abound in strategy analysis. For example, one future that was widely accepted to be true in healthcare in the 1990s was that capitation would be the predominant form of reimbursement in the future. Believing in this assumption, many organizations invested millions in primary care networks and integrated delivery systems. When capitation failed to materialize as expected, many organizations faced significant financial loses and their strategies had to be extensively revised or abandoned altogether.

What Is Scenario Analysis?

Scenario analysis offers a supplement or an alternative to the traditional one-future approaches to projecting and analyzing the future. Scenarios represent alternative constructed futures, but scenario analysis is not a process of generating multiple futures. It is a tool for fostering discussion, learning, and opening up to various eventualities. Scenarios thus facilitate more expansive thinking about the future; they offer a structured format within which the forces that might determine strategic success can be evaluated. Discussion of alternative scenarios allows management to deduce new patterns and trends and to form new mental models and theories. Scenarios should also challenge existing assumptions and preconceived notions about both the future and the strategies that might work.

Scenarios are literally small stories that are both plausible and believed to be important strategically. Although scenarios can be grounded in rigorous analysis, they should be highly creative. In fact, the scenarios that might best elicit thoughtful strategic thinking have characteristics of fairy tales, folktales, and even mythology. Scenarios are qualitative stories, written as narratives that typically describe the consequences for an organization given the conditions specified in each scenario setting. Such stories often have a psychological impact that traditional graphs and narrative plans do not; they help to explain why things happen by setting events within a constituent-focused context.

Typically, organizations create a small number of scenarios. Four scenarios, for example, are likely to be manageable but at the same time sufficient in number to elicit important possible future situations. Each of these would identify a different world and describe the organization's place within and strategic responses to each world.

The following are four possible themes for scenarios:

1. Scenario one: the world will be mostly the same as today only better
2. Scenario two: the world will be much better than today

3. Scenario three: the world will be mostly the same as today only worse

4. Scenario four: the world will be radically different from today

Alternatively, the scenarios can reflect particular trends, enabling specific consequences to be deduced. For example, if one believes that technology will significantly affect the future structuring of healthcare organizations (by affecting the degree to which integration of multiple facilities and provider groups can be accomplished with success, for example), then one might wish to evaluate one future where technology plays a major role and contrast this with another future where the scenario is different. The possibilities in the design of scenarios are only limited by the thoughtfulness and creativity of strategy analysts.

Constructing Scenarios

Scenarios can be constructed in various ways; one approach is described below.

1. *Define the scope and time frame for the scenarios.* The future time period that is appropriate for scenarios will depend on the speed with which factors considered to be important (e.g., technology, competitive practices, market structure, demographics) are likely to change. They will also reflect an organization's sense of its ability to respond to changes in its environment. Typically, a three- to five-year period would be appropriate in healthcare.

2. *Identify the key stakeholders who will be most interested in and affected by the scenarios.* Because scenarios are for strategy identification rather than strategy development, stakeholders such as customers or members at large might be invited to participate in the process.

3. *Identify the uncertainties that face the organization.* Here, a review of futurist imaginings and data analyses can be helpful. What are the potential uncertain challenges in the world that can affect your organization? What are predetermined environmental conditions? For example, although many insiders predicted capitation to become the primary form of reimbursement, the prediction was really an uncertainty, not a predetermined condition. On the other hand, many projections of demographic change are highly reliable and thus, in a sense, predetermined.

4. *Select the two most critical uncertainties.* One way to select the most critical is to rank the uncertainties by the degree of importance and

the possibility of their occurrence. Choose the two uncertainties that are expected to have the greatest impact (importance times probability) on the organization.

5. *Use the two key uncertainties to form the axes of a four-quadrant scenario matrix.*
6. *Name each of the four scenarios.* Use colorful, descriptive terms such as "Rose-Colored Glasses," "Death of a Profession," or "1,000 Flowers Bloom."
7. *Develop brief descriptions of their associated market conditions.*
8. *Ask the following questions to evaluate the appropriateness of the scenarios:*
   a. Do they bring forth fundamental strategic questions facing the organization?
   b. Does each represent a plausible future?
   c. Does each present fundamentally different futures and not just variations on a single theme?
   d. Do the scenarios challenge conventional wisdom?
9. *Discuss how choices today might affect the different futures.* What are the major resource allocation choices that arise, given the scenarios? How would shifts in resources affect the outcomes in each of the scenarios? Are there decisions that if taken would cripple the organization in any of the scenarios? Which scenario appears to be evolving or to be highly unpredictable? Implications for the organization should be clearly articulated and should be tied back to the organization's strategies.
10. *Identify road signs, trigger points, or markers that might alert the organization to shifts in the environment that can lead to a given scenario.* Such markers might be technology breakthroughs, changes in key legislation, structural change in the markets, or world events. For example, passage of a pharmaceutical benefit or discovery of a new biotechnology can move the world toward one of the devised scenarios.
11. *Establish a mechanism to monitor these road signs and periodically to update upper management on shifts in the environment.*

When incorporated effectively into the strategic analysis process, scenario planning can provide a valuable segue from the environmental assessment to the formation of strategic intent—the vision, goals, and values of the organization (see Chapter 3)—and the assessment of those strategies that will best ensure competitive advantage in an uncertain future.

Chapter 3

Strategic Intent

It is not cash that fuels the journey to the future, but the emotional and intellectual energy of every employee.... Yet if there is one conclusion to be drawn from the endless shifting of competitive fortunes it is this: Starting resource positions are a very poor predictor of future industry leadership.... Resourcefulness stems not from an elegantly structured strategic architecture, but from a deeply felt sense of purpose, a broadly shared dream, a truly seductive view of tomorrow's opportunity.... Strategic intent is our term for such an animating dream.

—*Hamel and Prahalad (1994, 139–42)* *

We hold these truths to be self-evident, that all men are created equal, that they are endowed by their Creator with certain inalienable Rights, that among these are Life, Liberty and the pursuit of Happiness.... That to secure these rights, Governments are instituted among Men, deriving their just powers from the consent of the governed.... That whenever any Form of Government becomes destructive of these ends, it is the Right of the People to alter or to abolish it, and to institute new Government, laying its foundation on such principles and organizing its powers in such form, as to them shall seem most likely to effect their Safety and Happiness.

—*from The Declaration of Independence, drafted by Thomas Jefferson and adopted by members of the Continental Congress on July 4, 1776*

IN THE ABOVE quote from the popular book *Competing for the Future*, authors Hamel and Prahalad (1994) suggest that the *strategic intent* of an organization, not its superior endowments of cash or other resources, is what drives its competitive engine. For Hamel and Prahalad, strategic intent is the "animating dream" that draws on the "emotional and intellectual energy" of organizational members to transform visions into winning reality. In this context, formalized strategies are the brains of competitive advantage; strategic intent is the heart.

According to Hamel and Prahalad, strategic intent motivates competitive strategy by providing organizations with three essential framing conditions: a sense of direction, a sense of discovery, and a sense of destiny. Strategic intent is directional in that it frames the ideas the organization needs to achieve its purposes. It is discovery in the sense that it provides the motive for organizational learning. It is destiny to the extent that the broader purposes of an organization are made explicit and an organization's strategies are designed to accomplish those purposes. All such functions of strategic intent serve to motivate employees, inspire creativity, and engender commitment to organizational goals and strategies. They all provide an institutional and moral frame within which the specifics of strategy are formulated.

Hamel and Prahalad's definition places the inspirational statements of organizations directly within the context of strategy; therefore, we apply it to three of the most important of such statements: values, mission, and vision. We suggest placing these three within a strategy context because to do otherwise is to relegate them to the land of platitudes. *Values, mission*, and *vision* take on particular utility when tied to decision-making processes that set the direction for an organization's growth and development—strategy.

This chapter addresses the interplay between the broader statements of organizational purpose and organizational strategy. The linkage between these is so important in healthcare because the industry operates within such a highly institutionalized and service-oriented environment. The issues involved in formulating strategic intent are explored with emphasis on statements of values, mission, and vision.

THE DEVELOPMENT OF STRATEGIC INTENT

The guiding concepts of values, mission, and vision are not new to the field of strategy. In fact, they have long been considered essential components of successful strategy making (Bennis and Namus 1985). These concepts (or statements, when operationalized) provide essential foresight and moral foundation, which help to move organizations beyond cold calculations about competitive maneuvering, financial return, or sources of advantage (Collins and Porras 1994).

A central problem inherent in constructing *strategic intent statements* is that they often devolve into mere exercises in institutional gesturing, characterized by wordy and lofty declarations that mostly decorate desks, hang on walls, and appear on web sites. As such, they often serve to placate external and internal stakeholders rather than light the way to an organization's future. Grand expressions of purpose, if not inculcated into an organization's culture, are unlikely to energize the organization or to play a meaningful role in shaping its strategies. Instead, they will appear more as "sounding brass, or a tinkling cymbal" (1 Corinthians 13:1) than as effective statements of strategic intent. Organizations do need to make explicit their principles, if for no other reason than to establish a moral context within which their actions and decisions are made. For those principles to serve this purpose, however, organizations need to move them beyond platitudes into tangible constructions of organizational purpose that actually shape, frame, and constrain strategic decision making.

Concreteness Versus Fluidity

Although the statements of strategic intent need to be grounded in enduring principles, they also should not be altogether unresponsive to changing environmental, market, and strategic conditions. On the one hand, they should provide a solid foundation for the rough and tumble of strategic decision making; on the other, if they are disassociated from current conditions, they risk becoming organizational gestures, designed more for public consumption than for use as decision-making guideposts. Clearly, a balance between stability and adaptability needs to be struck.

Valid, useful expressions of strategic intent will invariably contain some proprietary content; again, lacking such, they are likely to become more show than substance. Accordingly, portions of strategic intent possibly might not be widely shared beyond the walls of an organization, perhaps even beyond the offices of top management, while others will be broadcast openly and widely. Figure 3.1 arrays strategy and the statements of intent by the degree to which they are likely to contain proprietary content. Obviously, competitive strategies are highly proprietary and values are not.

Vision statements fall on the cusp between the purely inspirational and the strategic and proprietary. Therefore, statements of vision will likely vary from one organization to another by the degree to which they are intended to inspire and influence rather than to capture strategic purpose. They will also vary over time, as organizations adjust their sense of the future in the context of changing external and internal conditions. Vision statements are not the same as strategy, which are highly changeable and proprietary; rather, they are (or should be) reflective of the strategic environment. They thus should be adjusted occasionally if they are to remain relevant and current.

Who Should Formulate Strategic Intent?

The formulation of strategic intent should be a joint effort involving board members, management, and employees. This collaboration creates "buy in" and gives the statements their best chance of becoming embedded within the culture of the organization. That said, who in an organization

Figure 3.1. The Proprietary Spectrum of Strategic Intent

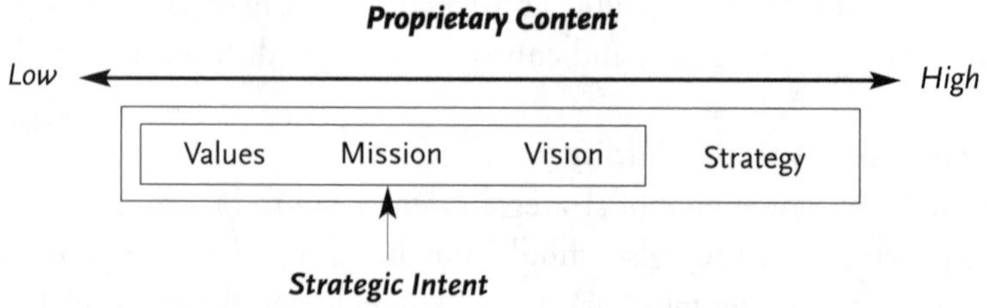

Proprietary Content

Low ⟵――――――――――――――――――――――――――――⟶ *High*

| Values | Mission | Vision | Strategy |

Strategic Intent

should take the initiative in formulating strategic intent remains to be determined. Several views on this exist.

One view suggests that management should take the lead, which presumably would increase the possibility that organizational purpose and strategy are integrated. Peter Drucker (1990, 5), one of the twentieth century's most prominent management authors, said, "The task of the...manager is to try to convert the organization's mission statement into specifics." These "specifics" include managerial daily actions in formulating organizational strategy. Giving the lead to management increases the prospects that these leaders will commit to the organization's purposes, thereby decreasing the likelihood that management only gives lip service to formulating strategy. Another view is that the board should take the initiating role (Pointer and Orlikoff 2002). By involving the board at the beginning of the process, the organization increases the possibility that the statements of purpose will reflect the interests of the organization's stakeholders and, possibly, even the community. It also increases the likelihood that those who oversee management will themselves be committed to the organization's general sense of direction.

Whichever of the two approaches is taken might be less important than ensuring that statements of purpose do not languish in organizational obscurity. Even the process of having management weigh in on the best ways to develop the statement can produce beneficial effects, drawing the attention of these leaders to the need to meaningfully link strategic intent to strategy.

Stakeholders and Legitimized Strategy

No business operates in a social vacuum. Each functions within complex composites of special interests, legal and regulatory frameworks, and conflicting value structures. An organization's strategic intent should fit firmly within these social constructs. Surely, the corporate scandals of 2001 and 2002 (e.g., Enron, WorldCom, Arthur Andersen, and National Century Financial Enterprises) are sufficient reminders of the obligations that business entities bear, obligations that are beyond those that emphasize profit making and overall organizational survival.

Healthcare providers especially, even those that are classified as for profit, have enduring societal expectations regarding their critical clinical responsibilities. These include duties to ensure that services delivered are appropriate and of a high quality, community needs are met, services are provided to the indigent and poor, research and education is supported, and so forth. In constructing and conforming to strategic intent, healthcare organizations should consider all such obligations and ensure that an appropriate balance is maintained among these obligations and, perhaps even more challenging, that strategic choices are compatible with them.

The external expectations placed on healthcare organizations are numerous, highly diverse, and often very powerful. Healthcare organizations perhaps face the most intense and complex array of externally generated pressures for social conformity of any industry in the United States. When actions do not conform to the bounds set by an organization's established intent, serious problems can arise. This occurs frequently in healthcare, for example, when organizations become myopically focused on profits or unyieldingly committed to specific strategies. By focusing inordinately on financial gain, for example, some not-for-profit organizations found themselves confronted by local and state governments intent on removing their tax status (see Strategy Note 3.1). Also, both not-for-profit and for-profit organizations, failing to attend to their values, have become the targets of governmental probes (see Strategy Note 3.2).

David Packard, cofounder of Hewlett-Packard Company, in 1960 expressed the need for a balanced focus between the public and the private financial interest of his company:

I want to discuss why a company exists in the first place. In other words, why are we here? I think many people assume, wrongly, that a company exists simply to make money. While this is an important result of a company's existence, we have to go deeper and find the real reasons for our being.... You look around and still see people who are interested in money and nothing else, but the underlying drives come largely from a desire to do something else—to make a product—to give a service—generally to do something which is of value. So with

> ## STRATEGY NOTE 3.1. UTAH CHALLENGES INTERMOUNTAIN HEALTH CARE ON TAX STATUS
> Source: *Modern Healthcare*, October 7, 1988, p. 12.
>
> In Utah, where the state Supreme Court ruled in 1987 that all not-for-profit hospitals must annually prove they deserve tax exemptions, four of nine not-for-profit hospitals and six ambulatory care clinics in Salt Lake County lost their tax exemptions and were told to pay a total of $2.4 million. Since those hearings, however, some not-for-profit providers have expanded charity care services and promoted their value to the community. The list includes two hospitals operated by Intermountain Health Care in Salt Lake City, which were denied tax exemptions. Pending appeal, none of the hospitals has paid its taxes.
>
> "We have made a greater effort to identify community need (since 1987)," said Douglas Hammer, Intermountain's general counsel. "We found it wasn't a case that people weren't getting the inpatient care they needed. It's more that there is a need for primary care, which has not been a role for hospitals in the past." In response, Intermountain now operates one "medically needy" indigent care clinic in Salt Lake County to serve a neighborhood where primary care was needed.

that in mind, let us discuss why the Hewlett-Packard Company exists.... The real reason for our existence is that we provide something which is unique. (Collins and Porras 1994, 56)

Constraints on Strategic Intent

Healthcare executives might need to go well beyond tinkering with the quality and acceptability of services to reconcile conflicts between the private and public interest. The challenge, however, is to balance their need for competitive advantage and financial viability against the diversity of expectations held by their many internal and external constituencies. Commonly referred to as *stakeholders* (Curry, Stark, and Summerhill 1999), these constituencies are individuals and organizations that have a stake or investment in and can influence the conduct and outcomes of healthcare organizations. Healthcare stakeholders range from patients to

STRATEGY NOTE 3.2. FOR-PROFIT COMPANIES AND COMMUNITY OBLIGATIONS

Source: Excerpted from Schinez, E. 1995. "From Scandal to Second Place." *Business Week* (November 27): 124.

Just two months after taking over at National Medical Enterprises Inc. (NME) in 1993, CEO Jeffrey C. Barbakow received a 7:30 a.m. phone call. Six hundred federal agents were rifling through records at NME's Santa Monica headquarters and at several of its psychiatric hospitals, in search for evidence of billing fraud and malpractice. By the time Barbakow arrived, a noisy phalanx of TV reporters was clustered in his office watching government workers roll out truckloads of documents. "It was a bad day," he says. "A complete mess." In the end, NME had to pay out more than a half-billion dollars to the government, insurance companies, and irate patients to clean up that mess.

Source: Excerpted from Eichenwald, K. 2000. "HCA to Pay $95 Million in Fraud Case." *New York Times* (December 15): section C, column 5, p. 1.

The nation's largest hospital company, which for much of a decade awed Wall Street with its ability to wring huge profits out of a once-staid industry, has agreed to pay $95 million in criminal penalties and plead guilty to charges that it obtained some of its money by cheating government health care programs, the Justice Department announced yesterday.... The settlement with the company, HCA–the Healthcare Company— formerly known as the Columbia/HCA Healthcare Corporation —is a partial resolution of sprawling criminal and civil investigations into its business practices. With yesterday's announcement, HCA has agreed to pay a total of $840 million in criminal and civil penalties so far this year. While that amounts to the largest fraud settlement in American history, large portions of the civil investigation are left to be resolved. In its criminal settlement, which is subject to approval by the courts, HCA will admit to submitting inflated bills and expenses to the government for reimbursement, illegally structuring business deals so that Medicare picked up the cost of corporate expenses, and providing doctors with kickbacks for patient referrals.

payers, from physicians to the community in general. Some exert little influence over healthcare organizations, but others are very powerful. All have expectations, rights, and responsibilities, even if these are not often made explicit or frequently expressed. Significantly, the number and power of stakeholders in healthcare have actually increased over the years, notably in direct proportion to increases in the efficacy and costs of care, both of which have risen precipitously over time (and they continue to rise).

Figure 3.2 shows that stakeholder interests individually and collectively form the institutional barriers that influence the actions and strategies of healthcare organizations. They moderate strategies from being "optimal," in terms of the strategies' potential to create advantage. The sum total of stakeholder impact is that they both legitimize and compromise strategies such that, to one degree or another, they become acceptable to, at least, the major stakeholders. Luke and Walston (2003) conceptualized institutional barriers as "intervening factors that shape and reshape strategic decisions consistent with institutional norms." These barriers prescribe the range of strategies that are, in effect, legitimate when viewed from the values and interests of diverse stakeholders. (The term "institutional" derives from the logic of institutional theory—see Strategy Note 3.3.)

The presence of institutional barriers might explain some of the otherwise inexplicable strategic moves taken by healthcare organizations, including the following:

- Catholic systems tend to merge only with other Catholic entities (see Chapter 8).
- Not-for-profit hospital systems avoid multimarket expansion (see Chapter 8).
- Many healthcare providers opt, at least initially, for the looser forms of organizational structure, rather than move directly into tightly controlled organizational forms or, conversely, jump prematurely to tightly controlled vertically integrated systems (see Chapter 10).
- Physicians are often able to resist management controls even when they are acquired by larger corporate entities.
- Academic medical centers encounter significant difficulties in merging with one another or being acquired by private companies.
- Significant resistance forms to for-profit system entry into markets in the Northeast and Midwest regions.
- Managed care companies face a backlash when they attempt to manage or control the costs of care.

Figure 3.2. Diverse Stakeholders Form Institutional Barriers and Legitimized Strategy

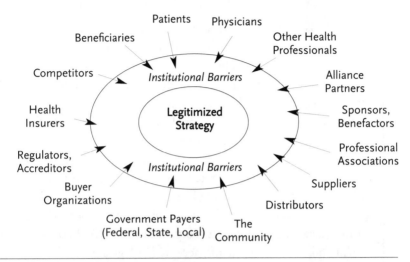

- Residual power is retained by many individual hospitals after being acquired by larger corporate entities.
- Vertical integration and portfolio strategies are avoided by provider organizations (see Chapter 7).

The above list could go on and on. The point is that stakeholders affect healthcare organizations' strategic intent in ways that can limit the organizations' ability to achieve strategic advantage. The organizations' values and interests thus circumscribe their range of strategic options.

The cloak of institutionalized influences (which represent only the tip of the influences iceberg) is particularly visible in the legal, regulatory, professional, and religious policies and procedures established within healthcare. Organizations need to recognize these constraints and work to balance them with their values, missions, visions, and strategies.

Formulating Strategic Intent

The legitimized values that emanate from stakeholders and the general environment are filtered through the formal expressions of an organization's ideals and aspirations: the statements of values, mission, and vision or the strategic intent. As expressed in Figure 3.3, these statements, presumably, shape and constrain the many decisions (both operational and strategic) that an organization makes.

STRATEGY NOTE 3.3. INSTITUTIONAL THEORY APPLIED TO HEALTHCARE

In the broader field of organizational theory, a specific theoretical framework—institutional theory—explains how sociopolitical forces affect the behaviors of otherwise rational organizations. Institutional theory suggests that organizational behaviors can be shaped as much by myth and irrationality as by established economic and organizational reasoning (Scott 1998). Such influences are said to be "institutionalized" in the environment—that is, they are deeply embedded within established belief systems and widely accepted as valid by many entities operating within an environment. The values from the institutional structure are well beyond the discretion of or the control by decision makers within individual organizations. As such, these values are taken for granted and accepted as legitimate.

In healthcare, such values are often established and reinforced through licensing, certification, payment, educational, ownership, sponsoring, regulatory, and many other processes and mechanisms. They inform all healthcare organizations of what they can and cannot do or should and should not do. The broad acceptance of such values and influences often leads to a behavioral pattern referred to as a "bandwagon" effect or as a form of "isomorphism." Under the bandwagon effect, rules are widely accepted, organizations comply with them and thus look alike, and, often, rationality is sacrificed in the pursuit of institutionalized legitimacy (DiMaggio and Powell 1983).

Scott (1998) suggested that healthcare is especially susceptible to institutional pressures and the pursuit of legitimacy. Throughout the 1990s, for example, healthcare providers consistently and universally adopted "faddish" structures and programs, most of which produced unrealistic expectations that ultimately were not often fulfilled. These included the legitimization of the so-called integrated system, acceptance of the strategic rationale for hospitals and/or physician practice management companies purchasing physician practices, and the ready adoption of "hot" management techniques (e.g., total quality management, reengineering, and corporate restructuring).

Figure 3.3. Determinants of Strategic Intent and Competitive Strategies

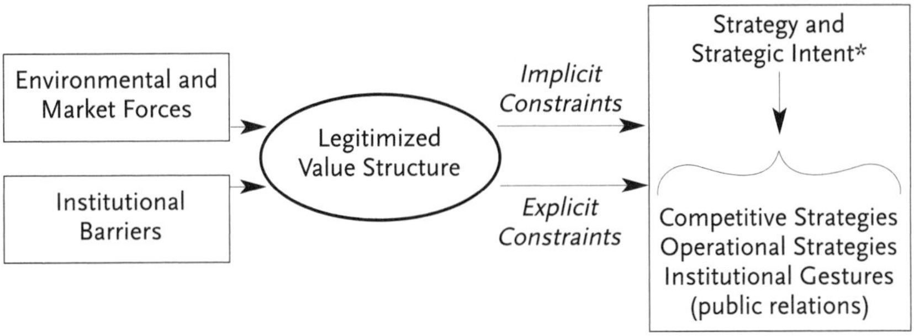

*Statements of an organization's values, mission, and vision

Each organization has slightly different value mixes and external influences. And each will use different filters through which to sort these values and influences and to determine their effects on organizational decision making. Different business models will therefore be associated with different statements of values, mission, and vision as well as different approaches to strategy. Varying business models are used especially in the hospital sector, where strategic intent and market strategies differ significantly. For example, a for-profit strategic intent and strategies are not the same as those of a not-for-profit's, a Catholic organization's differ from those of academic medical center's, a rural hospital's diverge from those of an urban hospital's, and so forth.

In the next section, we explore how meaningful statements of strategic intent are formulated and, more importantly, how they become an integral part of the strategies of organizations. We discuss the key role that management plays in providing leadership in the statements' definition and implementation.

VALUES

Perhaps more than any other document, the Declaration of Independence (see the quote at the beginning of the chapter) captures the strategic intent that continues to motivate American citizens to support their government and to pursue common national goals. The "self-evident truths" have become increasingly evident overtime, and they have provided the moral framework for most of this country's major (strategic and operational) decisions. Obviously, business organizations also need to be guided by shared and enduring values, a view clearly expressed by Thomas Watson, Jr. (1963, 3), former chairman of IBM:

> I believe that any organization, in order to survive and achieve success, must have a sound set of beliefs on which it premises all of its policies and actions.

On the other hand, in nearly every organization, certainly one or more employees have asked: "Is there really any value in articulating our values?" In general, employees may be in the best position to observe whether or not an organization's expressed values have been incorporated into its culture and strategies. In theory, organizational values represent the sum total of the individual values held by each person or stakeholders affiliated with an organization. In practice, however, the values of top executives almost always have the greatest influence on an organization's prevailing tone and practices. More generally, the CEO, other top executives, and the board are the ones responsible for formulating an organization's beliefs and preferences and promulgating those throughout the organization. Making certain that these beliefs and preferences are successfully inculcated within all parts of an organization and are fully embedded within its culture, however, is another matter.

A first step in this process is to formalize an organization's values in written statements. These written statements then serve as an ethical compass, providing direction to operational and strategic decision making. Lacking such a compass, an organization might experience a kind of *ethical drift*, where decisions lack measurable ethical standards. The possibility of ethical drift happening is greater during periods of environmental turbulence, at which times pressures to achieve financial and other performance-related goals can motivate individuals and groups to act in inappropriate or even unethical ways. Written values thus serve as visible reminders of the organization's commitment to basic beliefs.

Certainly, such reminders will be more effective if, in the process of their formulation and implementation, they have been carefully ingrained within the culture and structure of an organization. As a consultant once put it, "values written on a wall convey little, but these must be written in the hearts of employees to add worth." In Figure 3.4, we express the channels through which values, and the general elements of strategic intent, pass on their way to affecting market and operational strategies.

Figure 3.4. Decision-Making Flows and Feedback Between Strategic Intent and Competitive Strategy

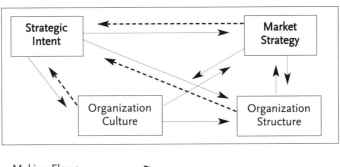

Decision-Making Flows ─────────▶
Feedback ‑ ‑ ‑ ‑ ‑ ‑ ‑ ‑▶

These values are a reflection of many externally legitimized values that are expressed both implicitly and explicitly. Some might come through formalized legal and regulatory structures, others out of the general environment that surrounds healthcare and the organization in particular. Those values affect strategies directly or in a filtered way through the organization's efforts to formulate strategic intent. In the figure, note that the solid arrows signify a direct effect and dashed arrows indirect effects.

As discussed in Chapter 1, strategy formulation is more a process than a one-time event. It is often incremental, so strategic options and logic change and evolve with organizational learning. Therefore, if values and other directional strategies have not been internalized within an organization, they stand little chance of affecting strategic and operational thinking over the long haul.

Failure to embed values also subjects an organization to the risk of *contingent ethics*—values that are acceptable in one situation but are irrelevant in another. Written values assist in grounding organizational ethics over time. Put another way, values and their companion ethics should endure, not fluctuate, through current encounters or challenges. Market strategies will (and should) change over time; values, generally, should not. On the other hand, as indicated in Figure 3.4, a feedback structure exists not only between strategy and statements of intent but also between culture and organizational structure and those statements. Although values should be relatively constant, they must be revisited from time to time for them to remain viable within an organization. Revisiting them would ensure that their mix remains consistent with how an organization might have evolved strategically over time. For example, a firm that moves into new markets might pick up new clients and powerful constituencies and thus might need to adjust its value mix and emphasis accordingly. For another example, a hospital system that integrates vertically into the business of managed care might face a significantly altered view of costs and its responsibilities for controlling these costs. Its values therefore might need to be adapted to this new strategic situation. Even without a major change in strategy or structure, an organization is likely to benefit by rethinking its values from time to time. At the very least, going through this process can help the organization recommit its members to the already-established values.

An especially important time for reassessing values is at the point of merger and acquisition. For example, when the Sisters of Charity Health Services (a Catholic system) combined with PorterCare Adventist Health System (an Adventist system) in 1996 forming Centura, both organizations had to adapt their original values to reflect the reality of their new strategic alliance. This undoubtedly was not a small task, not only because each organization had different religious beliefs but also because these organizations had been competitors in the Denver, Colorado, market for some time. All Saints Healthcare System, a multihospital system based in Racine, Wisconsin, is an organization that has a religiously grounded value statement; All Saints is also a member of the Wheaton Franciscan System, a larger Catholic multihospital system. Two of All Saints' expressed values are as follows:

Respect for the dignity of the individual.
We value each person as sacred, created in the image and likeness of God, which gives worth and meaning to each person's life.

Sharing with the poor.
We value sharing the gifts God has given us with those who are most in need and recognize the gifts we receive in return.

Assuming these All Saints values are inculcated within its culture, one should expect to observe that All Saints treats the poor with an added level of dignity. Furthermore, considerations of access and community needs should be visible, especially those that pertain to the location and types of service offered. The latter would be evidence that the organization's values are reflected in its decisions regarding strategic positioning.

Establishing Values

As mentioned, values should reflect the expectations of key shareholders. The following outlines one method by which this might be done:

- *Ask key stakeholders their desires for the organization.* In some organizations, the owners might be the only group truly deemed to be important. For others, multiple groups, including owners, customers, employees, and suppliers, might be influential enough to be included in a search for values. One way to identify key stakeholders is to identify those groups that would suffer most if the organization ceased to exist. Key stakeholders should be queried about the values they believe to be important. These questions can include "What do you want the organization to be known for?"; "What would make you proud to be affiliated with the organization?"; and "Where do you see the organization going, and why?"
- *Identify conflicting values among stakeholders.* Organizations should note those values that conflict between groups. If values conflict, the organization should prioritize the conflicting values and select those that are most closely aligned with the organization's purpose. Conflicting values might arise, for example, within a for-profit organization where investors place a particular emphasis on short-term profitability objectives while physicians value quality and investments in both information and clinical technologies, all of which can erode profits in the short term.
- *Create values that are distinctive.* Here, strategic intent interconnects with market strategies. To really make a difference, written values need to go beyond the bland, vague, or commonplace (for example, integrity and fairness). An organization might even choose values as a way to achieve some distinctiveness in the marketplace. In such cases, expressed values should make clear the underlying rationale and should provide a justifiable basis for differentiating the organization from its competitors. Statements of value should involve more than merely listing words (obviously, this is not easy to do); they should present evidence that these values can be and are being used. Also, they should be linked to measurable strategic outcomes, as reflected in satisfaction scores, error rates, availability of mental health care for homeless, and other such indicators. They can also be tied to organizational processes that are used to develop and implement strategic ideas.

All Saints is a good example of an organization that has attempted to go beyond merely listing its values—values that relate to wholeness, developing meaningful relationships with individuals and organizations, being good stewards of resources, and responding in times of special need. The organization did this by formulating some "Stand Fors" for its organizational actions and behaviors:

Our Stand Fors

Customer Relations
Make sure patients can schedule visits/admissions on a timely basis and in a convenient location; that the All Saints Healthcare "team" is supportive and caring of patients and visitors; that we retain a positive image in the community; that we are respected and preferred by payors; and that there is an internal culture of teamwork.

Physician Relations
Recruit and retain an appropriate number of physicians to meet the needs of the community while enhancing the practice environment of the Medical Staff.

Revenue Growth
Develop patient-centered approaches to All Saints Healthcare's growth.

Service Delivery Support
Continue to develop the support structure (such as leadership, information systems and facilities) required of a successful healthcare delivery system.

Sponsor Expectations
Meet our Wheaton Franciscan System sponsors' performance expectations in the areas of mission integration and Catholic identity, governance, spiritual care, ethics, human resources, and leadership development.

Strategic Financial Initiative
Implement identified activities that will support a positive bottom line within the balanced intent of all five goal statements.

All Saints values differ in some degree from those of other organizations and point to behaviors that can be assessed in terms of compliance.

The organization's values and stand fors, therefore, provide a good first step for All Saints as it seeks to tie these values to its pursuit of competitive advantage, at least in terms of improved positioning. All Saints stated values include some qualities that are commonly mentioned in value statements, such as honesty, integrity, leadership, teamwork, and fairness in all of their dealings. Yet, they also present some that are fairly distinctive, such as the development of employees, citizenship, duty and loyalty, and religious devotion.

MISSION AND VISION

Tying the mission and vision statements closely together is common practice (Quigley 1993). However, each serves two different purposes: missions express core purposes of the organization, and visions reflect where an organization wants to go, which ties it to strategy. A well thought out mission should express more than current purposes; it should also be forward looking. A mission statement can provide a conceptual bridge from the present to a desired and, hopefully, realistic future. (Many of the points developed in the following section apply as well to the formulation of vision statements.)

Mission Statements

1. *A mission statement should include measurable, definable, and actionable content.* In expressing an organization's purpose, a mission statement should be consistent with the organization's values and vision. Also, it should contain both product and market terms; the lack of either can disengage mission from strategy. Ask the following questions: What distinct products does the organization offer, and to whom? How does this mission differentiate the organization? Here is where the formation of mission should be integrated into the processes of strategy formulation. A mission statement such as "to care for patients" is relatively meaningless because it does not clarify the types of care or patients.

    Following is an example of an ambiguous mission statement of a large system: "to remain at the forefront of healthcare delivery." Although it is a laudable objective, this mission provides little indication as to what it means. Is the organization seeking to be in the forefront of clinical technology, market share, quality, or innovation? Here is another ambiguous statement: "providing healthcare services to the population of Company X's market area." Again, such a statement is too general. It provides no insight into what the organization aspires to become. Such statements, on the other hand, can serve a limited purpose of placating some external constituency. But it certainly does not provide sufficient content to marshal an organization's forces in the pursuit of specific strategic objectives.

2. *A mission statement should be compatible with the organization's strategic ideas (and vice versa).* A conflict between the mission and strategic idea, however, should not necessarily infer that the strategic idea is inappropriate. It can simply mean that the idea involves such a dramatic change that the mission no longer fits the path that the organization needs to take. In this case, the mission needs to be adjusted to accommodate the new direction. Therefore, although a mission should be relatively stable, it should not be immutable.

3. *A mission statement should distinguish the organization from others in its markets.* In the 1990s, hospitals were encouraged by their professional associations to incorporate a community benefit statement in their missions. Accordingly, the vast majority of hospital missions now include this information, which is reflected in the data gathered by the American Hospital Association (AHA). In its annual hospital survey, the AHA (2000) asks "Does the hospital's mission statement include a focus on community benefit?" By 1999, almost all (95 percent) hospitals responding to the survey reported that they included a focus on community benefit. This might be good from a public relations point of view, and it might serve to remind hospitals of the need to be responsive to their community's interest. But 95 percent compliance does not suggest that this community service statement is being used as a basis for product development, outreach policy, differentiation, or, least of all, strategy.

To be useful strategically, a mission needs to incorporate a defined, credible market, not one that is nondescript. The Scripps Clinic, located in San Diego, California, developed a statement that attempts to be somewhat more specific to its market:

> The mission of Scripps Clinic is to provide healthcare services of the highest possible quality to patients locally, nationally and internationally through a fully integrated, comprehensive healthcare delivery system.

This mission mentions three areas the company hopes to serve: local, national, and international. The latter two can be overreaching; on the other hand, Scripps, like a number of other highly respected and visible institutions (e.g., Mayo, The Cleveland Clinic, Methodist in Houston, Mount Sinai Hospital in New York, Shands) does draw patients nationally and internationally. The key is that Scripps, a prestigious delivery system, expresses the populations it intends to serve and has some success in serving.

By contrast, the mission of TriWest, a Phoenix, Arizona-based alliance owned by 11 Blue Cross plans and 2 university hospitals, is targeted to a more specific segment of the healthcare market:

> TriWest is committed to preserving the integrity, flexibility and durability of the military health care system by supplementing the military health care system with access to the finest health care services available, thereby contributing to the continued superiority of U.S. combat readiness.

TriWest confines its mission to one market segment, which imbues the statement with a degree of credibility.

4. *A mission statement should not be too restrictive.* During the early 1900s, the railroads in the United States fell on hard times because that industry narrowly defined its mission as providing rail service, rather than as being in the transportation business. The railroad companies remained committed to transportation on two rails, while much transportation shifted to roads and air. Likewise, hospitals that narrowly define their mission to be in the acute care business might encounter competitive difficulties in markets in which more integrated services are demanded. Such shifts in the environment might occur over the space of many years, even decades. Other changes might occur in a very short period of time, as was the case with many significant changes that took place in the 1990s. This reconfirms the need to reevaluate and update mission statements periodically.

5. *A mission statement should not contain strategically untested ideas.* This is perhaps the point at which missions and visions can be distinguished from one another. For example, a mission statement that directs a hospital to become an integrated delivery system, as

many did in the 1990s, might be venturing too much into uncharted or "visionary" waters. Given the rapidity of industry changes in that period, many provider organizations rushed to include such visionary ideas in their mission statements. In uncertain times, however, mission statements may be better off lagging behind rather than leading strategic ideas. Leading is the purview of the vision statement.

Another distinguishing quality between mission and vision is that the former is likely to be grounded in values and the latter in environmental assessments and strategic thinking. Including in a mission some untested strategic initiatives might draw the statement away from its key role: to articulate core values in a statement of purposes. Thus, an appropriate mission should be sufficiently descriptive to emphasize core organizational skills, but it should be broad enough to allow for creativity and innovation. This does not mean, on the other hand, that mission statements should not contain emphases on innovation. In fact, an organization is wise to express its role in adapting to changes in the environment. For example, Xerox has defined itself as "The Document Company" and its mission as follows:

> Our strategic intent is to help people find better ways to do great work—by constantly leading in document technologies, products and services that improve our customers' work processes and business results.

It is one thing for Xerox to say that it wishes to keep up with changing technologies and quite another to say that it is committed to a particular, even futuristic technology. The same holds for hospitals that express their intent to become integrated delivery systems when the validity of that particular idea remains untested.

Other companies have crafted more simplistic, yet effective, statements such as Honda's "beat GM!" Drucker (1994, 6–7) says that a mission should address "…your reason for being…" and "why do you do what you do." Yet a mission should not be a slogan nor should it be a strategic trial balloon. It should be a precise statement of established organizational purpose.

6. *A mission statement should reflect an organization's positive history and traditions, management preferences, distinctive competencies and resources, and existing or attainable competitive strengths.* To use effectively, a mission needs to be fully integrated with the actual activities

and competencies of the whole organization. It should reflect what the organization has done, what the organization's purpose for existing is, and for what the organization hopes to be remembered. For a mission to be effective, it must call individuals to action. It does this by

- eliciting an emotional, motivational response in employees
- being easily understood and transferable into daily individual action
- being a measurable, tangible goal
- being firmly rooted in the competitive environment in which the organization operates

Formulating Mission

No standard way exists for constructing missions. As with values, a mission is highly dependent on the input and direction of the organization's leadership. In consultation with the key stakeholders, leadership (board or management, depending on environmental conditions) can initially frame a mission, which should at minimum include the following:

- Product definition (e.g., "The Hospital Company")
- Standards and values to accomplish mission (e.g., "leading our industry in quality and service")
- Geographic market definition (e.g., "serving as a strong member of the Kitsap and Olympic Peninsulas' Healthcare System")

The following is a summary of the 14 steps in formulating a mission statement or reviewing or revising a current mission statement:

1. Establish a mission-writing group; this should be initiated by the chief executive officer. The group then performs the rest of the tasks below.
2. Make a list of the organization's core competencies and its unique strengths and weaknesses.
3. Make a list of the organization's primary customers by internal or external type, not by individual names.
4. Review each customer's requirements and desires for the organization. Develop a mechanism, such as a survey or focus group, for asking each key constituent group and for verifying the group's perceptions.

5. Write a one-sentence description of each customer's need-and-strength pairing.
6. Combine any descriptions that are essentially the same.
7. Pull out sentences of importance to the organization's mission, if one exists.
8. Combine the top three to five sentences into a paragraph.
9. Share the draft mission with the organization's customers. Ask if they want to do business with an organization that has such a mission.
10. Share the draft mission with employees. Determine if they understand and support it and can act on it.
11. Incorporate the feedback from customers and employees. If changes are needed, make such revisions and revert to step 8.
12. Identify changes that the organization has to make to fit in with the mission. Develop a plan of action to make these changes.
13. When the draft mission is refined into statements that clearly articulate the way the organization wants to relate to its constituencies, publish it, post it, and e-mail it to everyone.
14. Use the final (revised) mission statement to help in the formulation of the organization's strategies and actions. Critical decisions should reflect, support, and be tested against the mission statement.

After completion of a new or revised mission, the questions below might be used to evaluate the effectiveness of the mission:

1. Does the mission distinguish the organization from its competitors?
2. Is the mission too generic and not related to the value statement?
3. Does the mission express strategic intent?
   a. Does it help communicate a sense of direction and purpose to the employees?
   b. Is it used to drive decision making and resource allocation?
   c. Does it force managers to look for improvements to attain goals?
4. When was the last time someone referred to the values and mission of the organization while deliberating a decision?
5. What acceptable outcomes does the mission define? Are these measurable?
   a. Consider reputation, profits, effect on customers, community
   b. What mechanisms are structured to measure these outcomes?

6. Is the mission actually reflected in the organizational culture? How so?
   a. Are the things that are celebrated in the organization reflected in the intent of the mission?
   b. Do the business processes and personal and professional behaviors comply with the organization's mission?
   c. What are acceptable outcomes to reputation, profits, and effect on customers and community? Do these match the organization's mission?

In summary, a mission should direct the organization to focus its energies on certain products, standards, and market/geographic segments. The mission statement should be supported by the organizational culture and point to some of the ways by which the organization hopes to achieve competitive advantage. Missions that are consistently used in decision making eventually become part of the organizational culture.

Vision Statements

Pointer and Orlikoff (2002, 240) point out that vision statements play a far greater role in focusing on strategic ends than do statements of mission:

> Visions imagine the future, pointing to where an organization should go. Missions define the present, describing what an organization is. Visions challenge, missions anchor.

Moreover, vision statements serve a number of "core purposes" for an organization, purposes that Pointer and Orlikoff suggest should be articulated by the board and presented, in effect, to management as givens. (Pointer and Orlikoff clearly take the position that articulating strategic intent is the board's role.) Also, because of Pointer and Orlikoff's focus on the future, they suggest that visions should answer questions such as the following:

• Why should the organization exist, and what should it exist for?
• In what ways should it be different from what it is now?
• What should it not become? How should it remain the same?
• What must the organization do to advance the interests and meet the needs and expectations of key stakeholders?

- What type of clients should the organization serve? Whom should it be serving that it is not? What types of clients should it avoid?
- What types of benefits, services, and products should the organization provide?

A vision statement, as portrayed by Pointer and Orikoff, is closely aligned with proprietary strategy and thus helps to provide a general sense of direction. Such, for example, is contained in the vision of Tenet Healthcare, located in Santa Barbara, California:

> Tenet will distinguish itself as a leader in redefining health care delivery and will be recognized for the passion of its people and partners in providing quality, innovative care to the patients it serves in each community.

Two major factors that direct Tenet's strategy are the vision to be a leader in redefining healthcare delivery and the desire to have great passion for service. These should be helpful to Tenet leadership as they formulate their strategies.

Overall, mission and vision should be mutually supporting and direct the strategy of an organization. The creation of each should be done carefully to reflect proper values, but they should be succinct enough to be understandable and applicable. Both should be relatively stable over time (mission more so than vision), although as significant environmental conditions change, the organization should routinely reevaluate its mission and vision to align them with the changed environment and with the values and preferences of stakeholders.

Note: *Hamel and Pralahad quote on p. 59 is reprinted by permission of Harvard Business School Press. From *Competing for the Future* by G. Hamel and C. K. Pralahad. Boston, MA 1994. Copyright © 1994 by the Harvard Business School Publishing Corporation, all rights reserved.

CONCLUSION

This chapter discusses the importance and development of strategic intent, describing the elements of strategic intent—values, mission, and vision—and how these elements can be constrained by institutional pressures and should be integrated into the strategy-formulation processes.

Their formulation should also involve relevant stakeholders in an ongoing process, the outcome of which should be to create the moral and inspirational foundations on which strategies are built and implemented.

REFERENCES

American Hospital Association. 2000. *1999 American Hospital Association Annual Survey of Hospitals*. Chicago: Health Forum and American Hospital Association.

Bennis, W., and B. Namus. 1985. *Leaders: The Strategies for Taking Charge*. New York: Harper & Row.

Collins, J., and J. Porras. 1994. *Built to Last: Successful Habits of Visionary Companies*. New York: HarperCollins.

Curry, A., S. Stark, and L. Summerhill. 1999. "Patient Stakeholder Consultation in Healthcare." *Managing Service Quality* 9 (5): 327–36.

DiMaggio, P. J., and W. W. Powell. 1983. "The Iron Cage Revisited: Institutional Isomorphism and Collective Rationality in Organizational Fields." *American Sociological Review* 48 (2): 147–60.

Drucker, P. F. 1990. *Managing the Non-Profit Organization*. New York: Harper Business.

———. 1994. "Five Questions." *Executive Excellence* 11 (11): 6–7.

Eichenwald, K. 2000. "HCA to Pay $95 Million in Fraud Case." *New York Times* (December 15): section C, column 5, p. 1.

Hamel, G., and C. K. Prahalad. 1994. *Competing for the Future*. Boston: Harvard Business School Press.

Luke, R., and S. Walston. 2003. "Strategy in an Institutional Environment: Lessons Learned from the 90s 'Revolution' in Health Care." In *Advances in Health Care Organization Theory*, edited by S. Mick and M. Wyttenback. San Francisco: Jossey-Bass.

Modern Healthcare. 1988. "Utah Challenges Intermountain Health Care on Tax Status." *Modern Healthcare* (October 7): 12.

Pointer, D. D., and J. E. Orlikoff. 2002. *The High Performance Board: Principles of Nonprofit Organization Governance*. San Francisco: Jossey-Bass.

Quigley, J. V. 1993. *Vision: How Leaders Develop It, Share It, and Sustain It*. New York: McGraw-Hill.

Schinez, E. 1995. "From Scandal to Second Place." *Business Week* (November 27): 124–25.

Scott, W. R. 1998. *Organizations: Rational, Natural, and Open Systems*, 4th ed. Englewood Cliffs, NJ: Prentice-Hall.

Watson, T. J., Jr. 1963. *A Business and Its Beliefs*. New York: McGraw-Hill.

PART II

The Markets

Chapter 4

Market Structure

In the art of employing troops...do not fight on scattering terrain; do not stay on marginal terrain; do not attack the enemy on contested terrain; do not get cutoff on intermediate terrain; form alliances with the neighboring states at strategically vital intersections; plunder the enemy's resources on critical terrain; press ahead on difficult terrain; devise contingency plans on terrain vulnerable to ambush; and on terrain from which there is no way out, take the battle to the enemy.

—*Sun-Tzu (Carr 2000, 111 and 13)*

SUN TZU UNDERSTOOD that the strategies of war depend directly on the conditions under which the battles are waged. In the above quote, he identified nine types of terrain, each of which called for different approaches to strategy. In his writings, for example, Sun Tzu defined contested terrain as "Ground that gives us or the enemy the advantage in occupying it..." (Carr 2000). Obviously, if a battle centered on territory that is highly valuable to both sides, the intensity of the battle could be very great. Sun Tzu concluded that under such circumstances one should "not attack the enemy."

Market structure is the business strategy equivalent to Sun Tzu's concept of "terrain." In Chapter 2, we defined market structure as encompassing all of those institutional and organizational features of markets that shape the behaviors in which individual organizations engage as they seek competitive advantage over rivals. In this chapter, we develop the concept further and apply it to the analysis of strategy.

Just as the land on which a battle is fought conditions a war strategy, so too does market structure condition market competition strategy. For example, a hospital system competing in a relatively small and isolated market (the size of the market, which reflects both the number of competitors and the level of demand, is a general indicator of market structure) such as Merced, California, would likely pursue advantage in a very different way than if the system were competing in a large market such as San Francisco. Catholic Healthcare West (CHW) operates two acute care facilities in Merced, a metropolitan area with approximately 200,000 people. Together, the two hospitals control about 80 percent of the market. They face two small rivals in this market, one of which is owned by Sutter Health, a major player throughout the Northern California area but a small player in Merced. In San Francisco, by contrast, CHW operates 4 facilities (out of 19 in the market), which control only about 20 percent of the market. In the San Francisco market, Sutter Health is the leading player, owning six facilities that control around 30 percent of the market. Undoubtedly, CHW perceives the terrain in Merced (which is a much smaller market but one in which CHW has an unassailably dominant position) to be very different from that of San Francisco (a very large market in which CHW is in a tough competitive battle with two or three other major players). Accordingly, CHW's strategies should differ greatly between these two markets.

In this chapter, the conceptual foundations for the analysis of market structure are discussed. Some of the most important structural indicators are introduced, giving particular emphasis to market concentration and its measurement. Porter's (1980) widely recognized "five forces" model is examined, focusing on how the model applies directly to the analysis of healthcare markets, competitors, and organizational strategies. We present the stages of growth typology and explain how strategy is conditioned by the rate of growth in a market.

BASIC CONCEPTS OF MARKET STRUCTURE

Industrial organization (IO) economics serves as the intellectual foundations for the study of market structure. In Chapter 2, we pointed out that IO focuses much of its attention on public policy, especially on the use of antitrust enforcement to improve the performance of markets. Credit for applying the concepts and analytical frameworks of IO to the analysis of business strategy goes to Michael Porter, whose 1980 book, *Competitive Strategy*, has greatly influenced analytic thinking in the field of strategy. In this section, some of the key concepts of IO are introduced.

Specifying Markets

In textbooks on business strategy, "industry" rather than "market" commonly modifies "structure" or the two are used interchangeably. The reason is that these textbooks do not focus on any one industry and therefore contrast structural differences across industries. The automobile manufacturing industry, for example, might be shown to be more concentrated than, say, the retail grocery store industry. Our focus is on a single industry. Furthermore, our primary interest is in comparing markets within that industry.

"Industry" is often applied very broadly to healthcare—as in the healthcare industry. In this context, *healthcare industry* refers to all competitors engaged in the business of healthcare—namely, insurers, providers, and members of the supply-distribution channel. To avoid the confusion introduced by this common use of "industry," we use "sector" in the rest of this book when referring to subgroups within the broader healthcare industry—for example, the hospital, managed care, and physician sectors.

Even though "industry" and "market" are often used interchangeably, a clear distinction between the two should be made. *Industry* refers to the general collection of sellers whose products are close substitutes. *Markets* are specific; they include only those sellers that exchange with and compete for the patronage of the same group of buyers. In Chapter 2, we defined market as an arena in which one or more sellers of given products or services and their close substitutes compete for the patronage of and exchange with a group of buyers. The *arena* is the essential concept here. It refers either to a specific geographical area within which rivals compete or to a specific product type (e.g., emergency room services) or a category of products (e.g., acute care services) that are close substitutes for one another. Both geography and product are important in specifying market boundaries. Given the importance of spatial competition in the healthcare industry, the geographical definition is emphasized below.

Defining Markets by Geography

In the healthcare industry, especially in the provider and insurer sectors, competition and exchange occur within fairly well defined geographic areas. These areas are usually local, although they can be regional, national, and even international. (In this book, a local market refers to a metropolitan area; for nonurban competitors, to all rural areas within a given state.)

Many healthcare organizations compete within very small geographic areas. An individual hospital, for example, can compete only within a suburb of a metropolitan area. Some hospitals compete within and beyond metropolitan areas. Large referral centers can and often do provide services locally, regionally, nationally, and internationally. The prestigious Methodist Hospital in Houston, Texas, for example, serves mostly the local Houston market but also draws patients from many parts of the world.

How market boundaries are delineated, then, will depend on the purposes of analysis as well as the kinds of entities being examined. The Houston market provides a good case for demonstrating how an organization's purposes determine its choice of market boundary. If an organization were interested in studying Methodist's competitors in, say, hospital-based cardiac care, it might choose to examine rivalry within fairly narrowly defined geographic areas such as within individual zip codes or counties. Alternatively, if an organization were interested in acute care competition generally within Houston, it might define the market more broadly such as the whole Houston market; defining competitors more broadly might also be necessary. Thus, rather than examine competition for Methodist Hospital, the organization would more likely focus on Methodist's parent system in Houston—the Methodist Health Care System, which operates four hospitals in the Houston market. The competitors would then include many hospital clusters as well as freestanding hospitals such as Memorial Hermann (with eight hospitals), HCA (eight hospitals), Tenet (five hospitals), Harris County Hospital District (two hospitals), and St. Luke's Episcopal Health System (two hospitals).

If an organization wants to emphasize tertiary care, it might have to extend its market boundaries definition, restricting it to rivals that provide such services. At the tertiary care level, Methodist not only competes with two major referral centers located within the Texas Medical Center—Hermann Hospital (which is part of Memorial Hermann) and St. Luke's; it also competes with Baylor University Medical Center in Dallas, the University of Texas Medical Branch at Galveston, and other large and complex institutions in the state. On an international level, Methodist competes with a number of highly prestigious academic and referral centers, including Mayo, The Cleveland Clinic, New York Presbyterian, Orlando Regional, Johns Hopkins, and Scripps in San Diego. The point is that an organization needs to consider more than one market definition when studying competition.

The markets for supply-side organizations (manufacturers and distributors) in particular need to be examined at multiple levels. All distributors, for example, compete on the local level. In addition, the major competitors typically view their markets as broad regions. The leading distributors (big players) of medical-surgical supplies—McKesson, Cardinal, and Owens and Minor (the first two distribute pharmaceuticals as well)—compete with a number of smaller, regional distributors, but their primary threats come from one another as they battle locally and regionally for provider contracts across the country. The differences between the distribution and provider sectors highlight the need to be very clear not just about market boundaries (local, regional, national) but about which organizational units (local facility, local cluster of facilities, the company as a whole) or sectors of the industry (hospital, physician, managed care, supply distribution) are being analyzed.

Structural Measures and Market Boundaries

Misspecifications of boundaries and organizational definitions can lead to major errors in measuring market structure. For example, hospital market concentration measured broadly—say, at the regional level—is much lower than when measured narrowly such as at the local market level. This becomes clear when comparing the combined shares of the top four acute care hospital companies at the regional level against the summed shares of the top four at the local level. If measured at the regional level, the total market shares of the top four competitors in each region are as follows:

Northeast	13%
South	18%
Midwest	10%
West	22%

Contrast these percentages to 94 percent, which is the average for the top four hospital competitors per market, computed across all metropolitan areas. The numbers calculated by region suggest that the hospital sector is very fragmented, while the metropolitan figures suggest that it is highly concentrated. Which is correct? The latter, of course, more validly reflects hospital or hospital system markets (in this case, urban markets), in which rivals compete on a local basis.

Concentration measures (and other structural measures as well) also vary widely, depending on what facilities and services are included in the measures. If all types of hospitals (acute care general hospitals, specialty acute care hospitals, psychiatric hospitals, rehabilitation hospitals, long-term care facilities) were included in measuring concentration, then concentration would be lower than if the measurement were restricted to just one hospital type. The same holds for the services one chose to include in the measurement of concentration. One can study acute care hospitals generally or more specifically by type such as by examining only the cardiac services offered by acute care hospitals. Concentration in the latter case is likely much higher than was the general level of measurement used.

KEY DIMENSIONS OF MARKET STRUCTURE
Having discussed the problems inherent in specifying market boundaries, we turn to the major dimensions of market structure (Bain and Qualls 1987):

1. Degree of concentration
2. Height of entry barriers
3. Level of product differentiation in the market
4. Stage of market growth

In general, the greater the concentration, the higher the entry barriers; the more differentiated the products and competitors, the greater the market power each competitor will possess and the less price competitive the markets will be. Also, the slower the market growth, the more intense and threatening competition is likely to be; competition in no-growth situations effectively becomes a zero-sum game.

In the discussion to follow, we continue our emphasis on market concentration. We consider product differentiation specifically as a characteristic of monopolistically competitive markets and cover entry barriers and a number of other structural indicators when we examine Porter's five forces model. Market growth is discussed at the end of the chapter.

Market Concentration
Bain and Qualls (1987) derived the following typology of market models:

Atomistic Model: many competitors
- *Perfect Competition*: no product differentiation
- *Monopolistically Competitive*: product differentiation

Ogligopolistic Model: few competitors
- *No product differentiation*
    Easy entry

Moderately difficult entry
Blocked entry
- *Product differentiation*
Easy entry
Moderately difficult entry
Blocked entry

Monopolistic Model: one competitor.

Bain and Qualls structured their typology primarily around market concentration (although differentiation and entry barriers are used as well) because it is perhaps the most important structural feature of markets.

Atomistic Market Model

The *perfect competition* market assumes very low levels of concentration, low entry barriers, and no product differentiation. Competitors in such markets are thus assumed to have little or no market power—that is, they have little ability to set prices or to affect the competitive behaviors of their rivals. As a result, strategy for competitors in such markets would not likely focus on building power, either to countervail the moves of rivals (where the threat would be minimal) or to capture economies of large-scale organization (which by definition would not be present). Rather, competitors in perfect competition markets would be expected to turn their attention to building demand (positioning strategies) and controlling costs and internal processes and capabilities (potential and performance strategies) to maximize profits. Of course, few if any perfectly competitive markets exist. Thus, economists tend to relax one or more of the above assumptions to explore competition under real-world conditions. The consequence of this is that individual competitors are assumed to exercise market power. Removal of the large-numbers assumption, for example, means that individual competitors can be big enough to be capable of affecting prices and the strategic responses of their competitors.

Oligopolistic Market Model

Because of small numbers, competitors in oligopoly markets tend to be highly interdependent strategically, which is sometimes referred to as *conscious interdependence*. This means that competitors are often acutely aware that their survival depends on what their rivals do. A likely strategic response, therefore, would be to countervail the threats from rivals by engaging in acquisition and merger activities. Other market structure features condition the degree of threat an oligopolistic competitor might perceive. For example, if the barriers to entry are low, the consequent threat of entry can offset the concentrated power of a dominating rival, or high differentiation in a market can mitigate the harsh effects of oligopoly competition.

Because of high interdependencies, oligopoly competitors are likely to be relatively cautious when confronting rivals directly. Direct *price competition*, in particular, is often avoided in oligopoly markets because of the risk that such can lead to damaging price wars. This does not mean that oligopoly competitors do not engage in fierce competition with one another. On the contrary, they can be expected to pursue all forms of *nonprice competition*, which presumably are less likely to elicit damaging counter moves from rivals. Often, the first choice of oligopoly competitors is to pursue power strategies through merger and acquisition activities. Once consolidation opportunities have been exhausted, however, they are likely to turn to other nonprice options, which include investing in new product lines, increasing spending on advertising, focusing on quality and service orientations, seeking out distinctive locations, acquiring unique manpower and technologies, and signing exclusive contracts with buyers and sellers.

Hospitals, which are mostly in oligopolistic markets, appear to have been following this very sequence of strategic moves. In response to rising market threats, they pursued power strategies throughout the 1990s. But once such opportunities were diminished, at least at the local market level, these hospitals began to emphasize the great variety of nonprice options, which range from investing in information technologies to eliminating excess capacities. If competitive threats spike again, these hospitals likely will turn back to power strategies, this time possibly emphasizing multimarket as opposed to local market expansion (which refers mostly to the strategic responses of not-for-profit hospital systems; see Chapter 8).

Monopolistic Market Model

Large numbers of competitors combined with relatively high levels of product differentiation characterize monopolistically competitive markets. The corresponding relatively small sizes of competitors means that no one competitor has sufficient power to affect the well-being of the others. Lacking immediate threats from their rivals, competitors in such markets do not need to engage in the more aggressive forms of competition, especially price competition and power strategies. Instead, they focus on serving consumer needs (positioning), strengthening internal capabilities and resources, and improving performance.

Some competitors in fragmented markets might attempt to engage in power strategies, believing that market economics can sustain increases in market control and organizational scale. Such decisions are actually where the greatest opportunities and risks reside in monopolistically competitive markets. A competitor's success in uncovering the formula for consolidation produces an obvious advantage. The reverse, of course, is true if the competitor erred in its assumption that consolidation is possible.

This was the very calculation many physician practice management (PPM) organizations made in the 1990s. These PPMs assumed that the historically fragmented (monopolistically competitive) physician markets could successfully be consolidated. Much of their thinking relied on the assumption that successful contracting with managed care companies, integrating with hospital-based systems, and generally dealing with an increasingly complex market environment would make it necessary for physicians to practice in larger organizational forms. When most of their assumptions about the markets proved not to be true, the PPMs were left with having to extract advantages out of their practices by concentrating on improving practice efficiencies, which nearly universally failed to generate much advantage. A lesson learned from the PPM experience is that physician markets cannot profitably be consolidated, that they are inherently fragmented and will remain so for some time. On the other hand, the particulars of the PPM approach—outside organizations acquiring practices in multiple markets, bad strategic timing, poor implementation, poor assessments of the markets, poor choices of practice acquisitions, and too rapid growth—might have been the cause of the failure, not the idea of consolidation. In fact, the steady growth in the numbers and sizes of physician group practices in recent decades (Aventis 2001) suggests that the markets might be able to be consolidated, especially if physicians themselves, as opposed to distant corporate executives or local hospital administrators, were to initiate and manage the forming organizations.

Whether or not multimarket combinations will be attempted again in the physician sector may depend on future changes in the markets, such as a significant downturn in the economy and changing clinical technologies. In any case, perhaps the most important unanswered strategic question in the healthcare industry may be this: Are physician markets (which at this point in time are monopolistically competitive) capable of being consolidated?

Dual Economy Markets

Many markets actually combine the structural models discussed above. Sometimes called *dual* or *segmented markets* (Averitt 1968; Kanbur and McIntosh 1988), competitors in such markets face different structural worlds, depending on where they stand in the spectrum of market shares. In many oligopoly markets, for example, some competitors are so small (relative to the big players) that their market actions do not elicit strategic responses from larger competitors. These smaller competitors thus face very different market forces than do their larger, strategically more interdependent rivals. The smaller players thus tend to engage more in skirmishing for control over niches and other market residuals than confronting directly the larger rivals. In other words, they behave as if they are operating in a monopolistically competitive market structure, while their larger rivals compete in more oligopolistic environments.

Dual structures are actually fairly common in urban hospital markets, many of which are composed of a few large, very complex, dominating competitors and a fair number of smaller, less complex, peripheral players. Cleveland, Ohio, is a good example of a market that has a dual structure. As shown in Figure 4.1, the two top competitors—The Cleveland Clinic and the University Hospitals Health System—together control a total of 18 hospitals (representing 59 percent of the hospitals in the MSA [metropolitan statistical area]) and over 61 percent of the acute care patient days. The remaining 13 competitors each control one or two acute care facilities, totaling among them 16 hospitals in the market. Clearly, each of the two major competitors has sufficient market power to affect the other. Also, the differences in market power between these two and the others mean that no one of the smaller players is likely to be much of a threat to the big two. The smaller ones might threaten an individual hospital owned by one of the major players, but overall they would not likely appear on the strategic radar screens of the two big players. The smaller competitors, therefore, can be expected to operate within fairly well defined niches (in terms of geography or services offered) and to focus on consumer preferences (positioning), potential strategies, and performance improvements, which strategies are consistent with the responses of competitors in monopolistically competitive market structures.

Building on the Cleveland example, we contrast three categories of competitors often found in oligopolistically structured markets: *dominant organizations* (those with high and substantially greater shares than even their nearest rivals in terms of market share), *oligopoly groups* (small clus-

Figure 4.1. Competitor Categories, Using the Cleveland Market as an Example

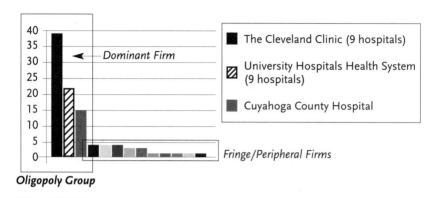

Oligopoly Group

ters of strong relatively equal competitors), and *fringe* or *peripheral companies* (smaller competitors each of which has very low shares). Dominance implies a form of market leadership in which most of the players tacitly accept and follow the lead role played by the dominant competitors. Markets that have dominant players provide little incentive for the remaining competitors to challenge them by engaging in further local merger and acquisition activities. Not all oligopoly markets contain each of these categories of competitors. As a result, they often differ in their competitiveness and degrees of stability (in terms of putting pressures on competitors to consolidate the markets even more).

Figure 4.2 displays three different distributions in market shares, one of which is characterized as unstable and the other two as relatively stable. In the figure, the Scranton, New Jersey, market, which is unstable, has a fairly long tail of peripheral competitors and lacks either a dominant player or a well-defined oligopoly group. Thus, Scranton appears to have good prospects for further consolidation, depending on many other factors such as cross-company incompatibilities and local market pressures. The other two markets are stable. The first—the Orlando market—is fairly evenly balanced between two large players and has only a minor fringe group in the market. Major shifts in power positions among any of these players is thus unlikely. The second—the Salt Lake City market—has a clear dominant player and a small oligopoly group. As a result, Salt Lake City offers little room for any of the players to restructure market shares. The competitors in this market are thus expected to turn to the other sources for advantage, rather than pursue local mergers and acquisitions.

Measuring Concentration

Two indicators of concentration are especially important:

1. The concentration ratio
2. The Herfindahl-Hirschman Index

The second is widely used in the arena of antitrust enforcement.

Concentration Ratio

The *concentration ratio* (CR) sums the market shares of some subset of top organizations in a market, which commonly includes the top four, although other numbers of competitors are used as well. The following is the general expression of the ratio (n equals the number of competitors):

$$CR_n = s_1 + s_2 + s_3 + \ldots + s_n$$

where s_1 is the market share of the ith competitor and n is the number of top competitors included in the measure (e.g., n = 4 for the four-firm ratio). CR values range from near zero (for highly fragmented markets) to near or equal to one (for tight oligopolies and monopolies). In general, the higher the value, the more concentrated and therefore the less price competitive the market.

Markets with four-firm ratios that measure 40 percent or less are commonly considered to be fragmented and thus assumed to be more price competitive. It is significant that only one hospital market falls in that range—Chicago, an MSA in which the top four organizations control around 36 percent of the market. Three other markets fall within the 40 to 50 percent range—Riverside, San Bernardino, California; Washington, DC; and Los Angeles. The remaining 327 urban hospital markets have CR measures above 50 percent. As mentioned earlier, the average for all urban markets is 94 percent, indicating a high degree of concentration at the local market level in the hospital sector. Virtually all nonurban markets (if measured at the level of individual towns) are either monopolies or have only a very few competitors.

The primary limitations of the *four-firm ratio* are that it does not include all competitors in the measure and includes no information about the distribution of shares among competitors. The share distributions can range very widely for markets that have the same four-firm ratio. For example, of just over 200 MSAs for which the ratio is 100 percent, the shares

Figure 4.2. Gradations in Shares Within and Stability of Markets

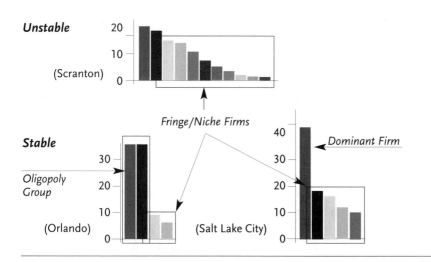

for the largest single competitor per market range from 100 (monopolies) to 29 percent. In other words, each of the markets in this group with four-firm ratios of 100 has the same measured level of concentration, but they vary significantly in their actual competitive structures.

Herfindahl-Hirschman Index

The *Herfindahl-Hirschman Index* (HHI) was designed not only to include all competitors but also to reflect the distribution in shares among them. HHI does this first by squaring each share and then summing these for all competitors in the market:

$$HHI = s_1^2 + s_2^2 + \ldots + s_n^2$$

where s_1 is the market share of the ith firm and n is the total number of competitors in the market.

The key feature of the HHI is the squaring of the shares, which serves to undervalue small shares and overvalue large ones, thereby magnifying concentration where it is extensive. Thus, for markets with the same number of competitors, the HHI is higher for those whose top one or two players have relatively high shares. Multiplying the HHI by 10,000 is a common practice that thereby effectively removes the decimal point. For example, an HHI of .4233 would be recorded as 4,233 after multiplying by 10,000.

The U.S. Department of Justice (2002) has established guidelines for judging levels of market concentration. Markets with HHI's under 1,000 are considered to have low concentration levels, those between 1,000 and 1,800 to be moderately concentrated, and those exceeding 1,800 to be highly concentrated and serious candidates for antitrust intervention. Only 6 urban hospital markets, or 2 percent, fall in the low concentration range; 31, or 9 percent, fall in the moderate concentration range; and 294, or 89 percent, are in the high concentration range. The average HHI across all urban markets is 4,727.

Limitations in Measuring Concentration

Both CR and HHI measures suffer from methodological limitations. First, they represent only one of many indicators of the presence of market power. Other indicators include the height of entry and/or exit barriers, degree of product differentiation, and presence of substitute products. For example, a market can appear to be concentrated only if competitors that produce the same product and are located within the same geographic market are evaluated. If, on the other hand, substitute products are important, such as ambulatory surgery centers, then not accounting in some way for these products can produce an overestimate of the actual level of concentration.

Second, how competitors are defined can make a significant difference in the measured shares and concentration. The Cleveland Clinic Hospital, for example, has a 16 percent share in Cleveland; but The Cleveland Clinic Health System, of which the hospital is a member, has a 39 percent share in that same market. The measurement of concentration at the hospital level (which is quite commonly done), rather than the local system level, understates concentration in markets in which considerable merger and acquisition activity has taken place. Deciding which form of competitor should be counted in the measures of concentration is also problematic. In the hospital sector, for example, many different types of hospitals (including children's, heart, cancer, women's, rehabilitation, and psychiatric) compete in the same markets alongside the more numerous acute care general and medical-surgical hospitals. Usually, comparing similar hospitals is important, which means specialty hospitals would be excluded when examining competition among more general hospitals and systems; this is the approach taken throughout this book. On the other hand, specialty hospitals do take market share away from general hospitals, even if only in a narrow band of services; this is a major problem that frequently arises in antitrust suits. Obviously, competitors that are under challenge for having built up too much monopoly power prefer a more liberal definition of competitors (which include specialty hospitals and substitutes) to ensure that measured levels of concentration are lower than they might otherwise be.

Third, aggregate indicators may not incorporate appropriate weights to account for the diversity of products that are often included in concentration measures. This is especially important when measuring hospital concentration because hospitals usually produce a wide range of services and operate different kinds of businesses. To a degree, the use of patient days does account for differences in the types of patients treated: presumably, sicker patients (e.g., cardiac care patients) stay longer than do others (e.g., pneumonia patients). For some purposes, additional corrections for intensity might be needed. Other such weights are the costs per case and indicators of case mix.

Fourth, concentration measures are highly sensitive to market size, especially for provider markets. Table 4.1 shows that measured levels of concentration for hospital markets are highly correlated with the size of the market, suggesting that in cross-sectional comparisons concentration measures are more likely to reflect differences in market size than in concentration. Further, the table shows that the two measures of hospital concentration—the HHI and the four-firm ratio—are more highly correlated with population size than with one another. Interestingly, the table also shows that the health maintenance organization (HMO) HHI is less correlated with market size than are the measures of hospital concentration. The correlations between the HMO HHI and the two hospital measures are even lower.

Because of the strong association between measures of hospital market concentration and market size, comparing hospital markets only within limited size ranges may be better. The value of doing this can be seen in Table 4.2, which displays markets that have populations between 1.5 and 3 million. In the table, the influence of population size is still apparent, but differences in the degree of concentration become clearer when observed within this narrower band of markets. Orlando (HHI = 0.37), for example, appears unmistakably to be more concentrated than Indianapolis (HHI = 0.17), both of which have similar population sizes.

Concentration in Healthcare Markets

As the foregoing discussion makes clear, hospital markets are highly oligopolistic; only a few would be classified as either low or moderately concentrated. Interestingly, the major buyer sector for hospitals—HMOs—has

Table 4.1. Correlations Between Market Size and Concentration Measures

	HMO HHI*	Hospital HHI	Hospital 4-Firm Ratio
HMO HHI	—		
Hospital HHI	0.40	—	
Hospital 4-Firm Ratio	0.39	0.62	—
Log Population	–0.52	–0.73	–0.80

*Herfindahl-Hirschman Index

also become highly concentrated. Table 4.3 compares the average hospital and HMO concentration measures for urban markets, controlling for population size. Relative to hospital markets, HMO markets are slightly more concentrated in larger urban markets and slightly less concentrated in smaller markets. Averaged over all urban markets, the HHI values are fairly similar—4,197 for HMO markets and 4,728 for hospital markets.

Although the managed care markets might exhibit near-equal levels of concentration to those of hospital markets, they likely differ considerably in the height of entry barriers (lower for managed care markets) and degrees of product differentiation (greater differentiation for hospital markets, due to location, plant age, medical staff, institutional affiliations, perceived levels of quality and service, and so forth). To the extent that this is true, hospitals should enjoy a competitive advantage over managed care companies. Of course, market power stems from other sources as well, including the overall size of the parent organizations, which typically favors the managed care companies. Concentration measures are not available for physician markets, but, as we suggested earlier, these markets are mostly monopolistically competitive. Physicians and their groups differ widely in their market characteristics (e.g., specialty, hospital affiliations, location, managed care contracts, group membership, reputations). Such differentiation gives many physician organizations considerable market power, despite their being relatively small in size and numerous within individual markets.

The markets for supply distribution are also highly concentrated. To some extent, the levels of concentration parallel those of hospitals and HMOs at the local level. Often, distributors sign contracts with provider organizations, which means they serve all hospital or physician members

Table 4.2. Concentration Between Similarly Sized Markets

Population[1]	MSA[2]	# of Competitors	HHI	4-Firm Ratio
2,968,806	Minneapolis–St. Paul, MN	16	0.17	0.68
2,846,289	Orange County, CA	14	0.16	0.71
2,813,833	San Diego, CA	13	0.14	0.67
2,753,913	Nassau–Suffolk, NY	13	0.20	0.74
2,603,607	St. Louis, MO–IL	21	0.13	0.62
2,552,994	Baltimore, MD	12	0.14	0.67
2,414,616	Seattle–Bellevue–Everett, WA	19	0.11	0.54
2,395,997	Tampa–St. Petersburg–Clearwater, FL	8	0.22	0.84
2,392,557	Oakland, CA	14	0.14	0.70
2,358,695	Pittsburgh, PA	23	0.14	0.61
2,253,362	Miami, FL	13	0.14	0.67
2,250,871	Cleveland–Lorain–Elyria, OH	15	0.23	0.80
2,109,282	Denver, CO	8	0.24	0.80
2,032,989	Newark, NJ	13	0.16	0.69
1,918,009	Portland–Vancouver, OR–WA	9	0.22	0.83
1,776,062	Kansas City, MO–KS	16	0.15	0.67
1,731,183	San Francisco	8	0.19	0.79
1,702,625	Fort Worth–Arlington, TX	10	0.18	0.70
1,682,585	San Jose, CA	8	0.19	0.71
1,646,395	Cincinnati, OH–KY–IN	7	0.28	0.94
1,644,561	Orlando, FL	4	0.37	1.00
1,628,197	Sacramento, CA	6	0.25	0.96
1,623,018	Fort Lauderdale, FL	6	0.20	0.87
1,607,486	Indianapolis, IN	14	0.17	0.76
1,592,383	San Antonio, TX	10	0.20	0.84
1,569,541	Norfolk–VA Beach–Newport News, VA	6	0.17	0.90
1,563,282	Las Vegas, NV–AZ	11	0.20	0.83
1,540,157	Columbus, OH	10	0.25	0.86
1,500,741	Milwaukee–Waukesha, WI	7	0.21	0.84

1. Population range is 1.5 to 3 million; 2. Metropolitan Statistical Area

within those companies locally. Also, distributors often sign contracts with more than one provider locally, which gives them even more clout at that level. On the other hand, despite the high levels of concentration and the absolute size of the big players (both Cardinal Health and

Table 4.3. Average Herfindahl-Hirshman Index, by Market Size

		Hospital Markets	*HMO Markets*
Market Size	250,000	6,533	5,208
	250 – <1 Million	3,930	3,980
	1 Million and >	1,903	2,219
	Overall	4,728	4,197

McKesson, the two largest distributors, are running around $40 billion in annual revenues), distributors are squeezed vertically between two strong sectors—the providers as buyers (whose market power stems mostly from local market concentration and differentiation) and the manufacturers as sellers. This and other structural characteristics tend to offset the dominant positions of the lead distributors, thereby heightening the overall level of competitiveness in their markets.

PORTER'S FIVE FORCES FRAMEWORK

Porter (1980) expanded considerably the structural elements that one might consider in assessing the competitiveness of markets for purposes of strategy analysis. In Table 4.4, some of these elements are presented using the categories identified in the five forces model, which is introduced in Chapter 2. Together, all of these contribute to the overall competitiveness of any given market.

Rival Threats

Rival threats are usually the most important of the five sources identified by Porter. Many structural features account for the intensity of threat. Big differences in the number of competitors, of course, are very important. Even within oligopolistically structured markets, small differences in the numbers of competitors can have significant consequences for overall levels of competitiveness. Few oligopoly competitors means that each rival is likely to be acutely aware of its interdependence with others and thus can be expected to restrain its strategic responses or avoid direct confrontation. By contrast, when there are more oligopoly competitors, some rivals might conclude that their strategic moves would go unnoticed and thus might be more willing to attempt aggressive maneuvers, including price competition.

For example, one can expect that competitors in the Houston market (which has 19 competitors composed of 45 hospitals, but 63 percent

Table 4.4. Structural Elements in Assessing Market Competitiveness

Rival Threats	Buyer Power	Substitute Products
Competitors • Numerous • Equally balanced • Diverse (ownership, business models) • Limited differentiation *Other threats* • High fixed costs • Lack switching costs • High strategic stakes • Slow industry growth • High exit barriers	• Market has few dominant buyers • Buyer has access to seller information; thus, buyer faces few switching costs and credible threat of backward integration • If buyer purchases undifferentiated products, buyer is unconstrained in switching sellers	• Result of rapid changes in technology, market structure, consumer preferences, and environment • Offer relative price • Present switching costs • Have buyer receptivity

Entry Barriers	Seller Power

Investment/cost barriers
• Economies of scale
• Capital requirements
• Switching costs
• Cost advantages:
  1. Distinctive resources/capabilities
  2. Product differentiation
Other barriers
• Legal restrictions (e.g. certificate-of-need laws)
• Institutional barriers
• Incumbent retaliation
	• Market has few dominant sellers
	• Seller has access to buyer information; thus, seller creates high switching costs and credible threat of forward integration
	• If seller sells differentiated products, buyer is constrained in switching sellers

of that market is controlled by the top 4 competitors) face a very different structure than do those in Denver (which has 8 competitors composed of 17 hospitals, but 80 percent of that market is controlled by the top 4 competitors). In Houston, there is much more room for maneuverability and a greater possibility for maverick strategic responses. Given the small number of competitors in Denver, strategic actions taken by anyone are not likely to go unnoticed by rivals. Relatively greater caution might therefore characterize the strategies of Denver-area competitors.

Other competitor characteristics are also important. The diversity in ownership or business models can be great across markets. Some competitors are owned by local systems and others by regionally or nationally distributed organizations. Some are for profit, others not for profit, and others Catholic. Some combine only small, community hospitals, while others configure hospitals into hub-spoke arrangements (see Chapter 8). If such diversity is high, competitors might have an inadequate understanding of the rationalities that drive their rivals and therefore can be tempted to make ill-advised moves that then trigger strong counter responses. On the other hand, dissimilar business models can tend toward niching, thereby increasing the stability of markets. For example, for-profit organizations can concentrate on the provision of basic services to suburban markets, and not for profits can emphasize the provision of higher levels of service to entire communities. Competitors might tend to pursue similar market segments in similar ways and therefore end up competing directly and aggressively with one another. In a related way, high differentiation can lead competitors to pursue different market segments and therefore reduce the overall level of rivalry in a market.

Many other factors influence patterns of rivalry, including a lack of switching costs (the costs that prevent buyers or sellers from disengaging from established exchange relationships), high strategic stakes (significant consequences that can result from the strategic moves in which they are engaged), slow industry growth, and high exit barriers. All such factors need to be carefully evaluated when assessing and comparing market structures.

Strategic Group Analysis

Given the importance of competitor diversity in assessing market competition, strategy analysts assign competitors to *strategic groups* based on the groups' distinctive approaches to achieving competitive advantage. Given their strategic commonalities, competitors within each group would then be assumed to respond in similar ways to market forces. Strategic group analysis is especially valuable in healthcare, given the wide diversity of competitor types (large/small, profit/not-for-profit) that operate in this industry. (Strategic group analysis is discussed here because it often draws heavily on market structure features and because it relates to assessment of Porter's rival threats.)

It is important to consider how difficult or easy it might be for members of one strategic group to attain the sources of advantage that distinguish the members of other groups. The degree of difficulty has been conceptualized as a *mobility barrier*. If the barrier is high, the members of one group are likely to experience difficulty duplicating the competitive advantages available to the members of another group. For example, the financial barriers preventing small, single-market multihospital systems from becoming large, multimarket systems is possibly very high. Or, widely dispersed hospital systems might find it difficult to restructure and begin capturing the advantages of tightly clustered systems (see Chapter 8 for further discussion of these model types). For example, Bon Secours, a Catholic multihospital system dispersed widely up and down the East Coast, is unlikely to be able to capture the advantages of a regionally clustered system such as Sutter Health System, the dominating regional competitor in the Northern California area.

Strategic grouping is also usefully applied to markets. In this case, markets would be grouped together if they shared similar market-structure characteristics. These *strategic market groups* (see Table 4.2 for an example) would be composed of markets that share the same structural characteristics and therefore can be assumed to shape the behaviors of competitors in similar ways. Strategic market group analysis is especially important in healthcare because of the importance and diversity of local markets in the industry. Strategic grouping, whether of competitors or markets, simplifies and enhances strategy analysis. It simplifies by reducing the numbers of factors that might be taken into account and by forcing the analyst to select those dimensions that might be of greatest importance to strategic success. It enhances by focusing the attention of the analyst on those examples across the country that might be most useful for making comparisons both within and between groups.

The analysis of a specific dominating, single-market hospital system, for example, might be greatly strengthened if the system's strategy were compared with those of other systems included in the same group. Such comparisons serve to highlight any subtle differences in strategy that might exist among same-group members. Between-group comparisons underscore uniqueness in strategic approach. Many analyses might also benefit from the combination of strategic group and strategic market group analyses. By controlling for market type (e.g., market size or region), comparisons between strategic competitor groups become more refined.

Identifying Dimensions for Analysis
The first step in strategic competitor or market group analyses is to identify the dimensions along which the competitors or markets might best be categorized. In the case of competitor analysis, the dimensions include any characteristic that might critically affect relative advantage and might enable clear distinctions to be drawn across groups. For example, hospital competitors might be grouped by the mix and structure of clinical services they offer, size or dispersion of the parent company, type of ownership, distinctive strategic approach (e.g., positioning, dominance, agility), specialization, rural or urban focus, and so forth.

Strategic group analysis can be applied to any of the healthcare sectors—hospitals, physician groups, managed care companies, distributors, and suppliers. In the managed care environment, for example, the predominant model used for structuring control over and payment to providers (e.g., group or staff models, preferred provider organizations [PPOs], independent practice associations [IPAs], networks) might be used. Physician competitors might be distinguished by the size of the group and by whether or not they are single or multimarket organizations. Distributors might be distinguished by whether they serve single or multimarket segments (including acute care, primary care, home health, long-term care, or all of these) or distribute single or multiple categories of products (e.g., medical/surgical supplies, pharmaceuticals, and major equipment, or all of these). The choice of dimension for grouping will clearly depend on the purposes of study and the particular competitors and markets being examined.

With regard to the grouping of markets, size is generally one of the variables considered. A small urban market, which has only a couple of competitors, differs significantly in terms of market dynamics from a market that has many competitors. (Los Angeles can hardly be considered in any way similar to Casper, Wyoming!) Other factors, of course, are also important:

- distinctive structural characteristics (e.g., concentration, rate of growth, degree of differentiation),
- distinctive healthcare characteristics such as managed care penetration and presence of certain types of competitors (e.g., for-profit competitors in the case of hospital markets),
- important geographical factors (e.g., urban or rural, region, the presence or absence of nearby rural and/or urban markets), and
- various population characteristics (e.g., population density, average income, population growth, percentage of minority in the population, percentage of aged).

The value of adding dimensions diminishes with the number of dimensions being used. One, two, or possibly three dimensions might productively be applied. Use of too many dimensions creates too many groups and introduces too many considerations for any useful insights to be gained. The key is for the analyst to conceptualize those particular competitor or market characteristics that most distinguish the members of one group from those in another.

Analyzing Business Units

The strategy analyst can find great value in conducting strategic group analyses of the multiple business units and diverse markets of larger organizations. This is similar to applying the Boston Consulting Group (BCG) Grid, except that the focus is not necessarily on the comparison of business units across different industries but on comparing business units or markets within the same industry.

We illustrate this application by examining the different market situations in which HCA, the largest multihospital company in the United States, has at least one acute care general hospital. In all, HCA is in 64 different urban markets and in a number of rural markets as well. Focusing on the urban markets only, a number of different dimensions can be used to classify the markets within which HCA is located. For example, one can use market growth (following the BCG Grid approach) or market size, which is one of the most important variables for differentiating market structures across local markets. Applying the latter variable to HCA, 36 percent of the organization's urban hospitals are in markets that are large (i.e., 1 million population or above); the remainder are in smaller markets. It is reasonable to expect that approaches to gaining competitive advantage are very different in large markets, such as Los Angeles, than in small markets, such as Boise, Idaho. HCA's urban hospitals and clusters also differ widely in the degree to which they are major players in their markets. For example, HCA's six-hospital cluster in Denver, which controls about a third of that market and is the leading competitor there, can be expected to engage in a very different form of competition than will its single (and small) hospitals located in Los Angeles and Washington, DC.

As shown in Figure 4.3, we apply these two dimensions—(1) market size (market characteristic) and (2) market share (business unit characteristic)—to illustrate the application of strategic grouping to the assessment of HCA's hospitals and local clusters in the urban markets in which HCA has facilities. Clearly, HCA's approach to strategy in the high market share/large market size situations should differ greatly from the strategic approach HCA might take in those large markets in which it has low market shares. In the latter, its strategies would likely focus more on niching, positioning, performance, and potential (discussed in Chapter 6); whereas in the former, the local HCA competitors might be expected to engage in all forms of power (discussed in chapters 7, 8, and 9) and nonprice competition.

In the smaller markets, the approaches to competition should also differ by relative market share. In those small markets in which HCA has a high market share (defined as exceeding 35 percent for small markets), HCA can be expected to function more like an oligopolist or monopolist (if the share approaches 100 percent), placing relatively greater emphasis on sustaining strong positions, erecting entry barriers, and so forth. In the small markets in which HCA has low market shares, HCA might be expected to focus on niching, positioning, or even getting out of the markets. Recall that in 2000, HCA spun off many hospitals in smaller markets, forming Triad and LifePoint (see Chapter 8). Perhaps HCA considered the small markets generally to offer few options for increasing advantage.

Entry Barriers

The height of *entry barriers* also can affect patterns of competition within markets. The lower the barriers, the more incumbent competitors need to worry about new rivals entering their markets and to be diligent about building sustainable competitive advantage. As shown in Table 4.4, entry barriers are attributable to either economic conditions in the market (e.g., economies of scale) or other sources (e.g., legal restrictions). Economic barriers are greater when high levels of one or more of the following exist:

- economies of scale;
- capital requirements;
- switching costs; and
- cost advantages such as new and efficient plants, distinctive resources/capabilities, and product differentiation.

All of these conditions are important in the various healthcare sectors.

Other sources of entry barriers identified in Table 4.4 should also be noted. Expansion in provider markets, for example, has been constrained by a variety of legal restrictions, such as certificate-of-need laws (which are present in about two-thirds of the states) or laws preventing the operation of for-profit entities (which is the situation, for example, in Minnesota). Certificate-of-need laws directly prevent expansions in capacity, whether by existing competitors or potential entrants. Both legal and economic sources of barriers place a high premium on mergers and acquisitions as a means for entry, rather than entry by expanding capacity.

One type of entry barrier that is especially distinctive to the provider sector is the presence of institutional barriers (see Chapter 3). Neither economics nor legal restrictions seem to explain, for example, many provider groups' (especially not-for-profit hospitals and systems) lack of movement toward multimarket strategies. A decrease in institutional barriers, on the

Figure 4.3. Typology of Market Groups for HCA's Urban Hospitals or Local Clusters

	Market Share[1]	
	High	Low
Large (1 million and >)	Richmond–Petersburg Austin–San Marcos Denver San Jose San Antonio Nashville Las Vegas Tampa–St. Petersburg Kansas City	Orlando Riverside–San Bernardino Atlanta Washington, DC Los Angeles–Long Beach Dallas Fort Lauderdale Fort Worth Houston Jacksonville Miami New Orleans Salt Lake City
Small[2] (< 1 million)	Fort Walton Beach Alexandria Fort Pierce–Port St. Lucie Corpus Christi El Paso Ocala Panama City Portsmouth Roanoke Terre Haute	Wilmington Lafayette Columbus Augusta–Aiken Boise City Lawrence Biloxi–Gulfport–Pascagoula Bronsville Olympia Provo–Orem Talahassee

Market Size (row axis label)

1. For large urban markets, a high market share is defined as exceeding 20 percent; for small markets, it is defined as exceeding 35 percent.
2. Only 11 of the 30 markets are included for small urban markets where HCA has low market shares

other hand, seems to explain why not-for-profit hospitals moved so aggressively in the 1990s to be part of multihospital combinations. Institutional barriers also might explain why most combinations in that decade were limited to local or regional combinations. Major discontinuities in strategy over time may be determined more by changing institutional conventions than by shifts in demand, technology, or the economics of production or system structuring. Finally, the threat of incumbent retaliation can be an important barrier to entry in many markets, especially in highly concentrated markets where individual competitors enjoy sufficient power to affect the success of rival entry. Incumbent retaliation is also likely to be a concern when incumbents have excess capacity (such as is generally true in the hospital sector) or highly flexible or liquid assets that can be marshaled in an attempt to prevent rival entry (see discussion of defense strategy in Chapter 5).

Barriers limiting the addition of new capacity have been low in the long-term care sector, where mostly for-profit entities enter local markets relatively freely and at small organizational scales. Entry barriers into managed care markets, whether by building new capacity or by acquisition, fell in the 1990s mostly as a result of an institutional sea change in which attitudes regarding managed care became much more accepting. Barriers to exit also have been and continue to be very low in managed care, which means that managed care companies move in and out of individual markets relatively rapidly (compared to the movement of provider organizations), and this has greatly intensified competition in managed care markets.

Buyer Power and Seller Power

Threats from *buyers and sellers* are discussed together given that one is essentially the inverse of the other. Competitive conflicts between buyers and sellers arise primarily in three areas. The first and most obvious area is the ongoing struggle between buyers and sellers over the prices and quantities of goods exchanged. The second area is more latent, but in selected circumstances it can be very serious: the threat that buyers and sellers pose to each other of backward or forward integration. The third is the power that both have to shift the balance of market power among their rivals. Such a shift can occur—for example, when a managed care company enters into an exclusive alliance with a local hospital system's most important rival, a move that would weaken that system while strengthening its rival.

The relative power enjoyed by buyers and sellers varies by the characteristics of the exchanging organizations and their products. As indicated in Table 4.4, buyer power is greater when only a few buyers dominate a market. Also, the more access that buyers have to the proprietary information of sellers, the fewer switching costs they face, and the more credible the threat that they will backward integrate, the greater the power they are likely to have over sellers. Similar but inverse relationships hold when viewed from the perspective of sellers. Buyer power is also associated with the characteristics of the products exchanged. If the products are undifferentiated, for example, the buyer will be relatively unconstrained in switching its seller. The same would be true if the products are less important to the success of the buyer in its markets.

Buyer-seller relationships, of course, can be and often are more cooperative than competitive. Interestingly, however, cooperation can have important strategic consequences unrelated to the explicit objectives of any cooperative arrangement. For example, in outsourcing the management, warehousing, and internal distribution of its medical-surgical supplies to its primary distributor, a healthcare provider can encounter serious switching costs that can later make changing distributors difficult. Under such an arrangement, the provider might need to adopt the distributor's proprietary information management system. In addition to the switching costs associated with such a move, the distributor also gains access to information that the hospital system might otherwise wish to keep confidential.

Both the buyers of healthcare services (managed care companies) and the sellers to providers (distributors and manufacturers) increased significantly their overall market power in recent years. Managed care organizations increased their penetration of individual markets. Distributors and manufacturers grew in size through a series of mergers and acquisitions. Neither, however, has been able to translate such gains into measurable additions in leverage over providers, especially over acute care providers. This is because hospitals effectively countervailed these moves when they formed into multihospital systems and local strategic clusters.

Another important countervailing move made by hospitals is that they joined powerful buyer groups, commonly referred to as group purchasing organizations (GPOs). Each of the two largest GPOs—Premier and Novation—represents between 1,500 and 2,400 hospitals. Together, they negotiate with suppliers on behalf of almost three-fourths of the hospitals in the United States. However, the GPOs do not own the hospital systems and thus have no direct power over these systems' actual product choices. The provider systems, in other words, are generally not obligated to make their purchases through the contracts negotiated by their GPOs. Furthermore, many systems are members of multiple GPOs; many enter into agreements with suppliers on their own; and few are able to effectively control their physicians and member hospitals, which often prefer products not covered by the GPO-negotiated contracts. As a result, the GPOs often struggle with the problem of compliance (the degree to which provider purchases are made through the contracted arrangements negotiated by their GPOs), which considerably weakens their clout over suppliers.

Substitutes

Substitutes can take two forms: (1) significantly different business models that compete in the same product areas and (2) distinctly different products that serve the same function from a consumer perspective. The latter form is the focus of Porter's five forces model (we discuss the former in Chapter 6).

Substitute products can be highly threatening to incumbent organizations for several reasons. First, substitutes can remain relatively invisible to incumbents until after they have begun influencing the market. This is because they often involve innovations of some sort, the importance of which might not be recognized right away by established competitors. Second, substitute products, if successfully introduced into the market, can potentially undermine the market value of established products. For this to happen, the substitutes must offer greater value in terms of preferred characteristics, lower prices, or both, which is a condition that is not easily accomplished because substitutes typically enter markets high up on the learning curve.

In the 1990s, substitutes played a key role in transforming the health insurance industry. In that decade, a variety of new managed care products (combined with new business models) rapidly displaced the once-dominant indemnity plans. The percentage of employees covered by indemnity insurance fell from 95 to 71 percent from 1978 to 1988, then it dropped precipitously to 14 percent by 1998 (Gabel et al. 2000). In the 1980s, dramatic changes in political, employer, and institutional environments played key roles in legitimizing managed care, which hastened the demise of indemnity products. Similar environmental changes, especially technological changes, stimulated substitute competition between traditionally in-house acute care and outpatient services.

Substitute products have been especially important in the surgical arena. As a consequence of improvements in both anesthetics and surgical procedures, outpatient surgeries now comprise over half (63 percent) of the surgeries performed in community hospitals in this country (National Center for Health Statistics 2002). Cardiovascular services have been especially susceptible to substitution. Cardiovascular-device companies have refined balloon angioplasty, radiation therapy, and minimally invasive procedures and have developed various medical technologies that enable once highly complex, in-hospital procedures to be performed outside the hospital surgical suite.

Hospitals, however, did not stand idly by watching the technological revolution threaten their markets. Instead, they embraced the new technologies, thereby transforming the battle from one of substitution to one of control. Hospitals used their considerable financial resources and system-building capabilities to capture and integrate many substitute services into their growing systems. The systems' sheer dominance at the local level gave them a significant advantage in competition with many upstart, substitute-providing companies.

The threat of substitutes remains high in the acute care sector, primarily because hospitals are such enticing targets. They are large, complex, costly, and preoccupied with many strategic and other challenges and threats. Specialty organizations can therefore be expected to find fertile ground in challenging hospitals, especially if they can move in rapidly, establish linkages with local providers, and convince consumers and payers of the greater value they offer. Continuing changes in technology coupled with rising costs ensure that substitution threats will persist in healthcare. Strategy analysts thus must remain vigilant in monitoring not only advancing technologies but also the emergence of businesses that seek to translate the new technologies into substitute products. Healthcare strategists need also to look inward to reassess their own systems of delivery and revisit otherwise sacrosanct assumptions about the structure and delivery of care. Also, they should establish a capability for change, which should include a supportive culture, good communications and relationships with both internal and external clinical constituencies, and financial reserve that can be directed toward new opportunities.

Healthcare is an industry overgrown with tradition and institutionalism, which together sustain an inordinate degree of myopia to new options and change. The environment, however, might no longer support organizational rigidity, inattentiveness, and institutional conformity. It might instead reward those systems that develop the capacity to adapt and reform.

STAGES OF MARKET GROWTH

The overall rate of growth is another market characteristic that should be considered when assessing the determinants of competition and strategy formation. The market stages model, originally applied to the study of product life cycles (see Figure 4.4), is undoubtedly the most widely recognized and useful conceptual scheme for studying the role of market growth (Kotler 1972).

In applying the market stages model to healthcare sectors, rather than to products, we hope to find out how the stages of market growth—emer-

Figure 4.4. Stages of Industry/Market Growth

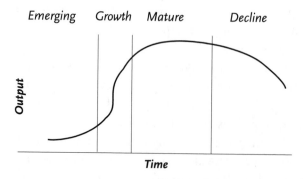

Source: Concept from Kotler, P. 1972. *Marketing Management*, 2nd ed. Englewood Cliffs, NJ: Prentice-Hall.

gent, growth, mature, and decline—affect the strategic behaviors of healthcare organizations and, as a possible consequence, alter the structural characteristics of their markets. We want to know how competitors in a mature market—say, those in the acute care sector—respond to the absence of growth, which is expected at the mature stage. Do the hospital competitors engage in intense rivalry because of stagnation in demand? Do they give added priority to controlling costs to compensate for slow growth in revenues? Of course, hospitals might do none of these things; this is because many other environmental and structural factors are at work, a point that reinforces the need for analysts to account for all of the relevant factors when studying market structure.

Not all markets flow through each of the stages, nor do they necessarily flow through them in the prescribed order. It would not be unusual, for example, for a market to reverse the expected sequence by shifting from a mature to a growth stage. A market can move into a period of decline and then, perhaps because of important demographic or technological shifts, change course and reenter a mature or even a growth stage. In fact, this latter possibility can easily happen (or may now be happening) in acute care, which has steadily lost ground as a result of substitutions of ambulatory for acute care services. Technological changes can allow acute care facilities to provide services in-house (or near by) in more cost-effective ways than possible in the past. The stages, therefore, should be seen as distinctive market conditions rather than as inevitable sequences through which all markets must pass.

Emergent Stage

Emerging markets characteristically experience high levels of uncertainty because of the newness of business models and market conditions. The *emergent stage* offers few clear rules to the game. The uncertainty stems from many factors, including the presence of new buyers and sellers; new products; evolving market structures; and, most importantly, changing technologies. Competitors in emerging markets are mostly embryonic—that is, they are usually small, new, and generally very high up on the learning curve. Diverse organizational types may be present in emerging markets; this is because proven approaches to competition may not have yet been established in the marketplace.

The key strategic imperatives in emerging markets are learning and pace (discussed in Chapter 5). Advantage most likely goes to competitors that are first in deducing the economics of the markets and then acting at the appropriate times. Environmental scanning is especially important for those initiating new products and businesses because such competitors easily become overly immersed in implementation and survival and fail to notice ongoing changes in the markets. The field of biotechnology provides a fertile ground for emerging markets because this is an area in which technology is exploding and its applications to healthcare are many but mostly untested. A wide range of diagnostic and therapeutic developments is available that hold out enormous prospects for revolutionizing healthcare. These developments include the following:

- new testing procedures that are noninvasive and provide near-immediate results;
- replacement genes that might treat some of the most deadly diseases;
- new vaccines that stimulate or suppress the immune system (suppressing organ transplant rejection, for example);
- regenerative medicine that might lead to the repair of injuries or reverse the effects of aging;
- stem cell therapies that can help combat illnesses such as diabetes, Parkinson's, Alzheimer's, and spinal cord injuries;
- modifications in microbial DNA to enable microbes to trigger antibody production; and
- genetic incorporation of vaccines into plants to help treat certain diseases.

Much of these advances are still being developed, but new technologies are being introduced to healthcare all the time. How the products of biotechnological research emerge within the systems for delivering care will be interesting to observe. Determining what kinds of organizations will dominate, whether economies of scale will prevail, how much niching will take place, and how high the entry and exit barriers will be, among others, will be important.

Growth Stage

The *growth stage*, by comparison to other phases, is relatively forgiving. Obviously, strategic errors made in good times are likely to be much less consequential than are mistakes made in no-growth environments. The intensity of rivalry also should be less in growth stage markets given that competitors in those markets have less pressure to grow by drawing demand away from rivals. Significant and long-run changes in the environment (e.g., changes in technology, emergence of new buyer segments, shifting entry and exit barriers) are generally needed for real transitions to occur among the stages. This might not apply so much to the growth stage, however, because growth ultimately is limited. As Porter (1980, 167) put it, "Eventually...an industry must reach essentially complete penetration. Its growth rate is then determined by replacement demand.... [Therefore] all very high growth rates eventually come to an end."

In many ways, therefore, growth stages are transitional; they are often relatively shorter in duration than are the other stages (as seen in Figure 4.4). Also, they can emerge at any time in the sequencing of the stages. Emergent, mature, even markets in decline can transition into a growth phase and then, after an appropriate period of time, move on to another stage. In fact, the acute care sector, which is commonly characterized as being in either a mature or a decline stage, might currently be moving into a protracted stage of growth as a result of the aging baby boomers, changing life expectancies, rising fertility rates, and other demographic trends (Solucient 2001). If so, strategies during such a period should consider not only how best to gain advantage during growth but also how best to prepare for whatever stage might follow thereafter.

Ambulatory surgery can be said to be in a growth stage. Innovative technologies continue to defuse into practice and established organizational modalities emerge. This is an especially interesting case because such growth in this area is often coupled with substitution threats for acute care.

Mature Stage

The *mature stage* is characterized by an overall slackening in demand, which can be very challenging for competitors. With limited expansion in demand, competitors discover that growth can be gained only by drawing market shares away from rivals. This typically leads to aggressive rivalry, especially in the early phases of market maturity. Being ill prepared for the slowing of growth, competitors easily make inaccurate assumptions about market conditions. Some might even add capacity, thinking that greater scale gives them an advantage. In fact, the management of capacity is a major strategic concern in the early phases of market maturity, as the hospital industry learned in the last several decades.

One can also find placid forms of competition in mature markets, especially once the early, often aggressive responses take their course and competitors come to accept a status quo. Having exhausted all viable options for direct confrontation, competitors often settle in and accept established positions among their rivals. Also, they often discover growth options outside their existing markets or businesses, which can transform them into multibusiness organizations. If the exit barriers are low and entry barriers are high, excess capacity can be driven out or new capacity can be prevented from entering, which also can contribute to a calming of market pressures in mature markets. Competitors in mature markets soon discover that the advantages of cooperation sometimes outweigh the costs and benefits of direct confrontation, which can increase the numbers of partnerships and other collaborative arrangements in the markets. As mature markets progress, therefore, competitors can be expected to shift their strategic priorities from growth to performance, from power to positioning, and from single-industry businesses to multiindustry businesses to compensate for the lack of opportunities to grow in traditional ways within mature markets.

Some of the above responses to changing market conditions were observed in the hospital sector in recent decades. The 1990s rush to consolidation, for example, can be viewed as a natural response to a maturing market (in combination with growing threats from buyers, the government, and other parties). The current emphasis on system refinements and integration is consistent with market maturity. Integration not only promises improved efficiencies but also opportunities for further growth through acquisition of non-acute-care businesses. The current emphasis on information systems, clinical management, organizational restructuring, reengineering, among others, might reflect a shift into a second refinement-focused phase within a mature hospital sector.

Decline Stage

The *decline stage* is difficult to identify because decline is not easy to recognize until it approaches the end phase. Also, decline can occur in some parts of a sector but not in others, making it difficult to draw overall conclusions about stages of growth. Decline can be rapid, as in the case where technological change is dramatic, or it can be gradual and protracted and possibly even imperceptible to most observers. For this reason, decline can easily be misinterpreted as a settling in of a mature market rather than the actual decline of that market.

The traditional prescription for decline is a harvest strategy, which refers to "eliminating investment and generating maximum cash flow from a business, followed by eventual divestment" (Porter 1980, 254). But this is not the only option available to competitors when markets are thought to be unhealthy. Porter identified four strategy options that competitors might adopt under conditions of decline:

1. Leadership: seek a dominant position in terms of market share
2. Niche: create or defend a strong position in a particular segment
3. Harvest: manage a controlled divestment
4. Divest quickly: liquidate and reinvest elsewhere

The *leadership strategy* assumes that dominance produces competitive advantage, especially if the decline is expected to be gradual. The *niche strategy* assumes that viable segments exist within declining markets that can be exploited successfully. The *harvest strategy* involves a gradual withdrawal of excess revenues or the selling of parts of a business over time. This strategy assumes that a gradual withdrawal would not cause undue harm to the business in the relative short term. If this were not a valid assumption, the *quick divestment strategy* might be the preferred option. This strategy aims to depart from the business while it is still financially viable to do so or, in more unfortunate circumstances, to withdraw when few choices remain.

CONCLUSION

The pursuit of competitive advantage must be analyzed in the context of important external forces; in this chapter, one of the most important external forces—market structure—is discussed. Very possibly the most important structural condition is the degree of market concentration. The number of competitors vying for limited demand can make a great difference in both the intensity of competition and the types of competition (sources of advantage pursued).

In recent decades, the healthcare industry went through a period of dramatic consolidation, thereby increasing significantly the overall level of concentration in many markets and markedly changing the dynamics of the markets. The implications of this change are critical for strategy analysts to understand. The analyst should also be fully aware of other important structural characteristics, including the heights of entry and exit barriers, the degree of product differentiation, the rate of market growth (or trend toward stagnation or decline), the power of various actors (including buyers, sellers, substitutes, and entrants), and other important characteristics of the markets.

In this chapter, we also explore strategic group analysis, which is simply a way by which markets or competitors can be compared within or between peer groups (the groups are defined by their similarities in competition and strategy characteristics). Comparing one's organization to other organizations that are in the same strategic group or those that are in different groups is important because it provides good insights into the nuances of differences among members of a strategic group. Comparison within one's market is also important. Strategic market and competitor group analyses highlight particular issues that the strategy analyst might otherwise not notice. This is especially important in the healthcare industry, where there is such diversity in business models, market threats, and market structures.

REFERENCES

Aventis. 2001. *Managed Care Digest* Series. [Online information; retrieved 1/03.] http://www.managedcaredigest.com/.

Averitt, R. T. 1968. *The Dual Economy: The Dynamics of American Industry Structure.* New York: W. W. Norton.

Bain, J. S., and D. Qualls. 1987. *Industrial Organization: A Treatise*, Volume 6, Part A. Greenwich, CT: JAI Press.

Carr, C., ed. 2000. "The Nine Kinds of Terrain," translated from Sun Tzu. In *The Book of War*, 111, 13. New York: Modern Library.

Gabel, J. R., P. B. Ginsburg, H. H. Whitmore, and J. D. Pickreign. 2000. "Withering on the Vine: The Decline of Indemnity Health Insurance." *Health Affairs* 19 (5): 152–57.

Kanbur, S. M. R., and J. McIntosh. 1988. "Dual Economy Models: Retrospect and Prospect." *Bulletin of Economic Research* 40 (2): 83–113.

Kotler, P. 1972. *Marketing Management*, 2nd ed. Englewood Cliffs, NJ: Prentice-Hall.

National Center for Health Statistics. 2002. *Health United States, 2002*. Hyattsville, MD: U.S. Department of Health and Human Services, Centers for Disease Control and Prevention, National Center for Health Statistics.

Porter, M. E. 1980. *Competitive Strategy*. New York: The Free Press.

Solucient. 2001. "National and Local Impact of Long-Term Demographic Change on Inpatient Acute Care: A Solucient White Paper." [Online article; retrieved 1/03.] http://www.solucient.com/publications/demochange.shtml.

U.S. Department of Justice. 2002. "Horizontal Guidelines." [Online information; retrieved 1/03.] http://www.usdoj.gov/atr/public/guidelines/horiz_book/toc.html.

PART III

Sources of Competitive Advantage

Chapter 5

Pace Strategies

By the end of the [19th] century artillery had undergone a transformation.... Some believed that the firepower of a larger number of attackers could overwhelm the defenders.... This defective reasoning contributed significantly to the emergence in European armies of a belief in the offensive.

—Jones (1987, 420–22).

A MAJOR MESSAGE in Jones's analysis of the art of war (see the above quote) is that many generals, from the days of the Romans to modern times, believed in the superiority of the offense over the defense. Unfortunately, this belief, especially if the offense is backed by a multitude of weapons and manpower, was present in World War I. In that war, the French, British, and other Allied commanders repeatedly took the offensive, sending hundreds of thousands of men to face the devastating defensive firepower of the well-dug-in German armies. Many lives might have been saved had the Allies known that innovations in technology had shifted the balance of power in favor of the defense, at least in land wars. This example is a painful reminder that overwhelming power might not be sufficient to secure advantage if the power is introduced in the wrong way or at the wrong moment.

Timing and the intensity of action—the essence of pace strategies—play important roles in producing competitive advantage. Too often, however, these are reduced to one-liner solutions or catchy clichés. The appeal to and need for organizations to be innovative, aggressive, visionary, and adaptable has spawned a host of articles, books, and consultants promoting one-dimensional formulations that suggest that complex and challenging strategic quandaries can be resolved simply by moving early.

Of the five major sources of advantage, pace is perhaps the most susceptible to oversimplification. Like the culture of the offensive that pervaded military thinking in the late nineteenth and early twentieth centuries, action orientations in the world of market strategy, if not carefully applied, easily disappoint in the unforgiving world of competition. Despite the plethora of ready answers, strategy analysts still must do the hard work of sorting through the haze of external and internal factors to determine how best to gain advantage in particular situations.

This chapter explores the conceptualizations and applications of pace as a source of competitive advantage. To provide the reader with a flavor for how pace is employed in strategy, a number of important concepts are explored, including hypercompetition, first-mover advantages, defense strategy, and the Miles and Snow typology.

PACE

Pace is perhaps the most tactical of the five sources of advantage because it deals with the punch and counterpunch of competition. It is concerned not just with timing but also with other action orientations such as the intensity of commitment, willingness to take risks, innovativeness and creativity, surprise, and the general aggressiveness with which strategy is pursued.

A clear predisposition toward action can be found in management and strategy literature. In their acclaimed book on corporate excellence, for example, Peters and Waterman (1982) identify eight essential attributes of excellence shared by the 75 major corporations the authors studied:

1. A bias for action
2. Close to the customer
3. Autonomy and entrepreneurship
4. Productivity through people
5. Hands on, value driven
6. Stick to the knitting
7. Simple form, lean staff
8. Simultaneous loose-tight properties

Not surprisingly, the first is a bias for action. Successful organizations, Peters and Waterman suggest, although good at analysis, are not constrained by the numbers or formulas comprising those analyses. Thus, these organizations tended to take opportunities before their rivals were prepared to do so. Other attributes of leading organizations also reflect an orientation toward action. The third in their list—autonomy and entrepreneurship—focuses on the need to encourage independent thinking and creativity, which are essential if an organization hopes to respond effectively and quickly to changing environmental circumstances. The last two—simple form, lean staff and simultaneous loose-tight properties—emphasize structures that have the greatest potential for fostering independent decision making and action. Again, these attributes reflect the perceived need for organizations to be nimble in the face of market and environmental turbulence.

In their book, Yoffie and Kwak (2001) draw analogies from judo to help explain organizations' need to be capable of taking quick, decisive, and unexpected actions in the marketplace. The authors applied the concepts of movement, balance, and leverage to strategy, all of which have to do with the action orientations that organization can take in the pursuit of advantage. Using judo principles, Yoffie and Kwak emphasize the need to produce the maximum impact with the least effort. Organizations, they suggest, should not pit strength against strength, but should use a rival's strength and size to throw it off balance and ultimately to gain competitive advantage. Building on these and other ideas, they offered a number of recommendations for organizations on how to compete using the principles of judo (see Table 5.1).

Regrettably, strategists such as Yoffie and Kwak tend not to highlight the significant risks that accompany aggressiveness in strategic maneuvering; they offer too much "feel good" in their prescriptions for action. The thrill of visualizing opportunities early and moving before rivals do, however, hardly counterbalances the many negative consequences that follow premature investments in unwarranted strategic actions. The list of organizations that failed because they moved too early and too aggressively is very long, including Enron outside of healthcare and Columbia/HCA within healthcare (in the 1990s). The 1990s produced many healthcare organizations that now wish they had exercised a bit more strategic caution, but the list of organizations that gained enormous success because they moved early is also very long. This includes Hill-Rom, an innovative company that because of early innovations and investments now dominates the bed and patient-support-system business serving the acute care sector.

Table 5.1. Judo Strategy: Approach to Gaining Competitve Advantage

Movement	Balance	Leverage
Don't Invite Attack • Keep a low profile • Position alongside competitors, instead of attacking head-on • Don't moon the giant *Define the Competitive Space* • Change the paradigm for redefining standards for the market • Segment the market and make focus the key • Use first-mover advantage to build market share *Follow Through Fast* • Stay focused and sequence growth • Make maintaining internal alignment an early priority • Use partnerships to leverage resources	*Grip Your Opponent* • Design joint ventures, etc., to co-opt or deflect the competition • Sell your services to opponents to stop them from developing competing capacities • Partner with opponents *Avoid Tit for Tat* • Avoid escalatory moves that drag you into a war of attrition • Study competitors carefully and copy only their most compelling ideas *Push When Pulled* • Find ways that allow you to use your competitor's moves to your advantage • Take the force out of your competitor's attack by building on his products, etc. • Don't fight losing battles: conserve your energy, fold your position, and return to fight	*Leverage Your Opponent's Assets* • Turn assets into hostages by forcing your opponents to cannibalize their own strengths to respond to your attack • Turn assets into handicaps that make it difficult for your opponents to compete • Execute, execute, execute—leverage is necessary, but not sufficient to win *Leverage Your Opponent's Partners* • Play on your opponent's partners' weakness to make it difficult for competitors to respond • Divide and conquer: force your opponents into unpleasant choices by pitting them against their partners *Leverage Your Opponent's Competitors* • Add value to your opponent's competitors' products • Create critical mass by building coalitions with your opponent's competitors • Provide a distribution channel for your opponent's competitors' products and services

Source: Concepts from Yoffie, D. B., and M. Kwak. 2001. *Judo Strategy: Turning Your Competitors' Strength to Your Advantage*. Boston: Harvard Business School Press.

Environmental Turbulence

The rise in interest in pace-related thinking in the strategy field is closely tied to changes in the environment and markets and, more particularly, to the speed with which those changes are occurring. Various forces are commonly identified, but the most fundamental of these is technological change. With the advent of computers, telecommunications, and the Internet, so the argument goes, markets now change far more rapidly and organizations need to be much more adaptive than in the past. Other trends have also contributed to the importance of pace as a possible source of advantage, including the rise in global competition, shifts in demography, alterations in consumer preferences, changes in the patterns of competition, and the emergence of new types of competitors. All of these trends are important strategically because they increase the prospect of strategic surprise or "sudden, urgent, unfamiliar changes," as Ansoff referred to them (1977, 55). With the possible exception of global competition, these trends are also important in healthcare.

In addition to such broad trends in the environment, other forces can cause competitors to worry more than usual about timing, risk taking, and other pace-related orientations. Abrupt changes in market structure, whatever their causes, can precipitate unplanned strategic maneuvering. A fall in entry barriers, for example, can introduce into markets not only new competitors but also different business models and types of products (especially, substitutes). Such changes were clearly important in healthcare in the 1990s; they permanently altered the competitive dynamics of many once-stable markets.

The key point to remember is that action orientations are closely tied to environmental and market structure conditions and changes. In stable markets, organizations might not need to move aggressively and take on added risks. In turbulent environments, by contrast, vigilance and readiness to alter strategies offer the potential for creating real advantages. On the other hand, aggressive actions taken in times of uncertainty can be much riskier than when pursued in stable market conditions. Therefore, organizational leaders must actively monitor their markets and environments and prepare their organizations to take critical strategic decisions if such are merited. Also, leaders must be capable of assessing the risks of either action or inaction. The key here is readiness—to be prepared for action when required in changing markets and environmental conditions—not action per se.

Hypercompetition

In his book on *hypercompetition*, D'Aveni (1994) presents an interesting conceptualization of how strategy should change amid significant environmental turbulence. In the face of rapid technological innovation, D'Aveni argues, know-how is more easily transferred and acquired, entry barriers are no longer the stabilizing force, and deep pockets no longer provide the protection against competitive threat. Organizations thus must shift their strategic directions more quickly and frequently under such conditions if they hope to ensure profitability within so-called hypercompetitive markets. To be hypercompetitive, however, market change has to be both significant and continuous. Temporary shocks or bursts of competitive activity do not constitute hypercompetition, no matter how dramatic such a change is. Technological change, in particular, can produce conditions consistent with hypercompetition; such changes can continue for extended periods of time, as witnessed by the ongoing revolution in information and other technologies. Technology can also play a facilitating role, enabling organizations to move rapidly and unpredictably to enter new markets, create unique business models, and offer novel products and services.

Under hypercompetitive conditions, D'Aveni states that organizations should not "stick to the knitting" or focus single-mindedly on sustaining existing sources of advantage. Established sources of advantage might quickly become obsolete under these conditions. Thus, organizations should actively engage in the search for new advantages while allowing established advantages to be eroded, which will likely happen despite an organization's best efforts to the contrary. As a result of this, organizations should drastically shorten their time horizons. As soon as they achieve some profitability, they should begin looking for other sources of advantage and enable existing advantages to be eroded, as D'Aveni (1994, 8–11) put it:

> So what is the harm of trying to sustain an advantage for as long as possible? In an environment in which advantages are rapidly eroding, sustaining advantages can be a distraction from developing new ones. It is like shoveling sand against the tide rather than moving on to higher ground .... The primary goal...is disruption of the status quo, to seize the initiative through creating a series of temporary advantages .... Strategies such as "stick to the knitting" and "build off your core competence" may maximize short-run performance and profitability

by using the same assets over and over again. But these approaches do not provide…for true long-run survival. While they may generate short-term profits, these strategies ultimately leave companies with a tired, out-dated asset base that is not adapting to the future."

Based on D'Aveni's logic, we suggest that the central objective should be to sustain established sources of competitive advantage rather than to ensure profitability (see Figure 5.1). Under normal conditions, one might expect a considerable amount of time to pass not only before rivals mount serious counter moves but also before established advantages are effectively eroded and new sources have to be identified. In hypercompetitive environments, on the other hand, the whole time frame is condensed. The lag preceding competitor attack, the duration of sustainable advantage, and the time available to establish new advantages are all shortened. Also, the intensity of advantage is reduced because so much less time is available to build and extract a return from established advantages. Under such conditions, the strategist needs to be diligent in assessing competitor threats and trends and new opportunities for building advantage.

D'Aveni boiled down to seven the strategies—he called these the New Seven Ss—that organizations need to take under conditions of hypercompetition:

1. Superior **stakeholder satisfaction**
2. Strategic **soothsaying**
3. Positioning for **speed**
4. Positioning for **surprise**
5. **Shifting** the rules of competition
6. **Signaling** strategic intent
7. Simultaneous and sequential **strategic thrusts**

D'Aveni added the the term "new" to distinguish his recommendations from McKinsey's seven Ss (Waterman, Peters, and Phillips 1980). The first S—stakeholder satisfaction—is a reminder of the significance of bringing one's stakeholders along when change comes about unexpectedly and rapidly. The next three—soothsaying, speed, and surprise—are unique capabilities that organizations need to move successfully with greater pace. The last three—shifting the rules, signaling, and simultaneous and sequential thrusts—are pace-related tactics that organizations are expected to take to throw competitors off balance in a rapidly changing environment. Of course, all of these Ss presuppose that hypercompetitive conditions actually exist, that these conditions contribute to patterns of rapid erosion in the sources of competitive advantage, and that new sources of advantage can readily be identified. Of course, it is possible that none of these conditions holds or occurs simultaneously. A hypercompetitive environment depends on significant and ongoing changes in technology, with continuing periods of innovation and obsolescence. As the dot-com bust and the concurrent overinvestments in information technologies demonstrate so clearly, it is very easy to overestimate the importance and impacts of technology on organizational performance or, more particularly, on the need to adopt new strategies.

Hypercompetition in Healthcare
The healthcare industry experienced an extended period of unprecedented change in the 1990s, but did that constitute a form of hypercompetition as conceived by D'Aveni? To those on the firing line, it might have appeared to be hypercompetitive. One-time upheavals, however, do not constitute hypercompetition.

In the 1990s, payment and market structures changed dramatically at the same time. Perhaps the most significant and disruptive change was that many markets shifted from fragmented to consolidated states (see Figure 5.2). This shift and other important changes in that period were undoubtedly highly destabilizing. Metaphorically, healthcare experienced the equivalent of an earthquake, the consequences (aftershocks) of which are still ongoing. But the primary shock is over; it was a one-time event and, as a result, the post-1990s environment is much calmer, even though the new restructuring remains intact and continues to evolve gradually. Unexpected, continuing changes will likely occur in the future, and such events can produce important strategic surprises. But, again, hypercompetition by definition involves extended periods of ongoing instability and change in which organizations need to be highly and continuously focused on visioning, speed, adaptability, and the search for new sources of competitive advantage.

The real value of thinking about hypercompetition is that it reminds us that there are times when organizations need to be more adaptive than they had been in the past. They might need to build new sources of advantage and to give up on the old. The danger at such times is that many organizations lack the essential capabilities for change and their cultures might not accommodate change, even when new approaches are obviously

Figure 5.1. Lifecycle of Competitive Advantage: Traditional Versus Hypercompetitive Environments

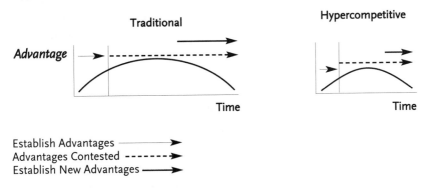

Source: Adapted with the permission of The Free Press, a Division of Simon & Schuster Adult Publishing Group, from HYPERCOMPETITION: Managing the Dynamics of Strategic Maneuvering by Richard A. D'Aveni. Copyright © 1994 by Richard D'Aveni.

needed. Once again, developing a capacity and a readiness for change is crucial, even if only limited actions are taken ultimately, a point that is consistent with the arguments of both Peters and Waterman and Yoffie and Kwak.

STRATEGIC ORIENTATION

A few concepts relating to pace have become standards in healthcare. Some of the more common pace-related terms include adaptability (Chakravarthy 1982); flexibility (Harrigan 1985); surprise (Rothschild 1984); initiative (MacMillan 1984); learning (Mintzberg 1978); and defense (Porter 1980). To further illustrate the concept of pace as an orientation to strategy, three pace-related concepts are discussed in this chapter: first-mover advantages and the experience curve, defense strategy, and the Miles and Snow typology of strategic orientations.

First-Mover Advantage

First-mover advantage is perhaps the most recognized pace concept in the literature. Broadly promulgated in the mid-1960s by the Boston Consulting Group, the assumption is that first movers, by being first, are capable of achieving dominating positions in their markets (see Henderson 1979). However, despite long-held assumptions about the inherent advantages of first movers or pioneer organizations, research evidence has been mixed in showing that this advantage actually bears out in practice (see Lieberman and Montgomery 1998). The rationale for first movers remains strong, however. Among the most important arguments supporting this concept is that, with time and experience, organizations are able to refine their administrative and production processes and thereby move steadily down the average cost curve for their particular industries. This gives such organizations considerable advantages over later movers, which are assumed to enter at the same high point on the cost curves at which the first movers had entered and therefore be at a considerable strategic disadvantage. The advantages of first movers, in fact, can be overwhelming, with Microsoft as a prime example. Invention, however, is often the key to such advantages, suggesting that significant early moving advantages in healthcare are likely to be found in the supply and manufacturing sector where the possibilities for new product development are great more than in the retail or delivery and payment sides of the industry. This does not mean, however, that many provider or managed care organizations will not gain first-mover advantages; it only means that such advantages might likely come from innovative business models than from the development of overwhelmingly successful product lines.

If first or early movers gain access to superior resources and capabilities, they can use these to erect entry or mobility barriers, thereby blocking entry or deterring strategic moves by others. Such resources might include access to patents, better locations, and superior manpower. With these resources, early movers can expand product lines and engender superior recognition, commitment, and switching costs in the consuming public. Also, first movers likely can capture economies of scale and scope (multiproduct or multibusiness economies) before late entrants are able to do so. On the other hand, early movers might not be able to sustain the lead implied by their *experience curve*. Later movers or entrants might, for example, be able to piggyback on, learn from, or imitate the experiences of the early mover, giving them the capability of moving in at a much lower level of cost than otherwise expected. In addition, there is the risk that the first mover has not yet discovered the best ways to do things. Having taken action in the earliest phases of market development, early movers might have failed to access the best resources and technologies given that these resources might not have been visible, known, or even available in the early stages. Thus, early movers risk committing to resources and capabilities that, as competition proceeds, prove inadequate or obsolete. Further, some presumed advantages simply might not

Figure 5.2. Market Restructuring in Healthcare

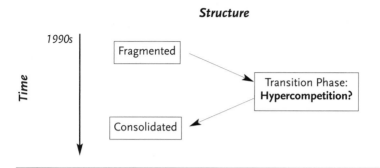

be easy to sustain; for example, superior manpower can be recruited away by later movers. Late movers also face risks. The most obvious is that, by waiting, they risk preemption by early movers. Early movers can erect barriers that make competing on equal grounds difficult or even possible for followers. Also, late movers simply risk being blindsided, not having anticipated the defensive moves of an early mover or the consequences of such moves.

The evidence (most of which is anecdotal) supporting early mover advantages in healthcare is not even. Several healthcare organizations—Intermountain Healthcare in Salt Lake City, Utah; Sutter in Sacramento, California; and Sentara in Norfolk, Virginia (all of which moved into multihospital forms and invested aggressively in other healthcare businesses before it was fashionable for not-for profit organizations to do so)—appear to have gained considerable advantages as early movers. They have built highly successful, complex delivery systems that are widely considered to be among the best in the United States. However, a number of high-profile organizations have not been successful with early moving; such high-profile examples as Columbia/HCA, Phycor, and Medpartners come to mind. For these specific organizations, the failure appears to come from experimentation, specifically with efforts to consolidate to a degree that the structural capacity of their markets could not sustain.

Defense Strategies

Defense strategies are mostly preemptive. They differ from offense strategies in that their objective is to decrease the chances and possible impacts of an attack. Defense strategies are not focused on creating competitive advantage but on sustaining it. As such, they can be very costly, providing benefits only in the long run, if at all. Therefore, a defense strategy must be as carefully considered as would any other strategy pursued by an organization. Much of the discussion of defense strategy focuses on preventing entry. However, we generalize the concept by applying it to the prevention of any strategic move of either a potential entrant or an existing rival. The key to defense is not only to anticipate a strategic attack but also to conceive of the sequence of steps through which the attack might pass as it is implemented, as Porter (1985, 483) put it:

> The formulation of defense strategy must begin by recognizing that an attack…is a time-phased sequence of decisions and actions. Appropriate defensive strategy must be formulated in the context of the entire assault, and not just one move.

As illustrated in Figure 5.3, defense strategy deals with preventing strategic moves and attacking a rival after a move has been initiated. Efforts to deter come at the earliest point, before any move is made. This is the most general and diffuse defensive response and thus possibly the most costly to execute. In such cases, the total costs of defense might never be known because costs can be embedded within many functional and daily activities carried out by defense-oriented organizations. At the stage of deterrence, a rival does not know with any certainty from what direction or at what time a competitor move might come. Obviously, not every move can be anticipated or defended against; thus, a premium at this stage is on intelligence gathering and on erecting structural barriers to possible strategic moves; put another way, an ounce of carefully placed prevention might be worth a pound of cure.

Deterrence can continue once a rival's move is detected; here, defense becomes much more focused, although the emphasis remains on deterring or inhibiting that move. Once a rival move is well underway, it is likely to pass through various steps; here, the challenge of the strategist is to focus on those steps, creating counter moves as appropriate. Then comes the stage at which the move is completed; here, defense strategy is much less distinguishable from offense strategy. Defense blends into offense as time progresses.

Porter discussed a number of possible defense moves that competitors might need to execute, some of which are listed in Table 5.2. A tactic commonly employed by healthcare providers is to fill product or positioning gaps by broadening product lines or closing off niches. Healthcare organizations often try to anticipate the service options that rivals might

Figure 5.3. Stages in Defense Strategy

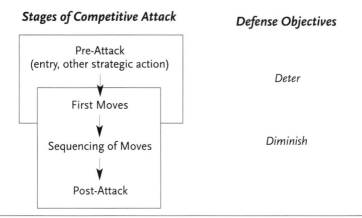

Stages of Competitive Attack   *Defense Objectives*

Pre-Attack
(entry, other strategic action)

Deter

First Moves

Sequencing of Moves   *Diminish*

Post-Attack

pursue and then fill those gaps before rivals or new entrants are able to do so. Signaling is another important strategic tactic that might not be utilized in healthcare to the degree possible. A provider might signal its intentions to enter a market or develop a product line well before it actually plans to make such a move. For the signal to have a deterrence effect, however, it must be credible; if not backed by recognized cash reserves or excess production capacity, a strategic signal might not be taken seriously. A competitor needs to make it clear that it is truly committed to a signaled move. Rivals also can evaluate intentions to follow through by referencing a rival's history in following through with action after signaling its intentions. On the other hand, public announcements of intentions can carry considerable weight. The announcement of future products (vaporware, for example), even when they are still in early stages of development, is a highly successful and frequently utilized defense strategy in the software business.

The strategic move taken by Carilion Health System based in Roanoke, Virginia, provides an example of a defense strategy. One might quibble about whether Carilion's strategic decisions were offensive or defensive, but the effect of those decisions has deterred rivals from moving into Carilion's territory. In its earlier years, Roanoke Memorial Hospital (the initiating hospital that created Carilion) faced threats not just from rivals in its own market but from those located within an hour or less from Roanoke. To shore up its position in the local market, Roanoke Memorial Hospital first acquired the only other not-for-profit hospital in town, Roanoke Community Hospital. The acquisition measurably strengthened Carilion's position in Roanoke (the combined entities now control about

Table 5.2. Some Defense Tactics

Raise Structural Barriers
- Fill product or positioning gaps (e.g., broadening product lines, closing off niches)
- Block channel access (through use of exclusive agreements)
- Raise buyer switching costs
- Increase scale economics/input costs
- Build interrelationships (through use of alliances)
- Encourage government's restrictive policies

Increase Expected Retaliation
- Signal
  1. Commitment to defend (e.g., announce intentions to build capacity)
  2. Incipient barriers (e.g., new planned products, technological changes)
- Accumulate retaliatory "war chest"
  1. Set example for action (build credibility)
  2. Establish defensive coalitions

Source: Concepts from Porter, M. 1985. *Competitive Advantage: Creating and Sustaining Superior Performance*. New York: The Free Press.

---

two-thirds to three-fourths of the local acute care market) and prevented (a defensive objective) the HCA rival in town, Lewis Gale Medical Center, from capturing Roanoke Community Hospital. This example illustrates the high overlap that often exists between offense and defense strategies; Carilion's moves clearly combine both. More importantly, a defensive move that does not involve some offense (which carries some clear source of immediate gain in advantage) can be costly.

Carilion also sought to shore up its position against more distant rivals—two-hospital Centra Health, Inc., located about 35 miles away in Lynchburg, and University of Virginia Health System, located in Charlottesville. As a defensive move, Carilion acquired or secured management contracts with eight nearby nonurban hospitals. Had Carilion not done this, those hospitals could have been captured by one of Carilion's distant rivals. Recently, Carilion entered into an agreement with Lynchburg-based Centra Health to jointly own and operate the rural Bedford Memorial Hospital (now renamed as a Carilion hospital); it has also entered into joint ventures with University of Virginia Health System as well. Carilion was able to take these moves because of the strong defensive position it has attained. This string of acquisitions and co-opting moves has undoubtedly helped Carilion block many incursions that might have been made by its nearby rivals.

The Carilion example is fairly representative of many acquisitions, especially local acquisition, accomplished by hospitals in the 1990s. At that time, a number of hospitals feared that if they did not move, rivals would beat them to the punch and thereby strengthen their own positions within the local markets.

Miles and Snow Typology

Nearly 20 years ago, Raymond Miles and Charles Snow (1978) constructed one of the most interesting and widely recognized typologies of pace strategies. Specifically, they identified four strategic patterns that differ from one another by the degree to which an organization's leaders are willing to assume risk or take aggressive action in the pursuit of competitive advantage. The four model types are as follows:

1. Prospector: organizations that frequently search for new market opportunities and regularly engage in experimentation and innovation
2. Analyzer: organizations that maintain stable operations in some areas but also search for new opportunities, often following the lead of prospector organizations
3. Defender: organizations that rely on established approaches to growth and seldom make adjustments to existing, proven strategies
4. Reactor: organizations that perceive opportunities and turbulence but are not able to adapt consistently or effectively

The *prospector* orientation is the most interesting of the four because of its emphasis on aggressive market and product development. Thus, given their more aggressive strategic orientations, prospectors are most likely to adapt successfully, or at least more quickly, to situations in which the environment is turbulent and uncertain. However, prospectors are also more likely to fail given that new, aggressive business ventures and maneuvers are associated with high rates of failure. In the 1980s, for example, Humana (which became the first major acquisition of Columbia during its dramatic growth in the early 1990s) was consistently among the first to pursue new business ventures: for example, it invested in the "doc in the box" concept, a convenience strategy that did not catch on in the industry at that time. Humana was also a leader in developing centers of excellence in multiple sites. In the 1980s, it was a major sponsor of the Jarvik Heart (artificial heart) and the experimental surgeries performed by Dr. William DeVries. Also, Humana invested heavily in a managed care company, which it attempted to integrate vertically with its second largest multihospital company (see Chapter 9). Both Humana in the 1980s and Columbia/HCA in the 1990s experienced significant growth, but both experienced significant failures in some of their aggressive strategic efforts.

At the other end of the spectrum is the *defender* orientation, which responds to environmental threats in ways that are effectively the opposite of the prospector's. The defender turns inward, seeking to buffer its business activities from external challenge. The defender can be aggressive, but more in defending its turf rather than in expanding products or entering new markets. In effect, the defender builds its competitive advantages though positioning, performance, and potential (see Chapter 6). More than do other orientations, the defender invests in technology and emphasizes efficiencies. Unlike the prospector, the defender tends to be narrower in product and market diversity. The strategically conservative orientation of the defender means that it will do well in stable environments. Under conditions of environmental turbulence, however, the defender fails to respond adequately or in sufficient time when needed. Alternatively, of course, it can avoid the mistakes made by rivals that overreact to temporary or misunderstood environmental change. An excellent example of this orientation is Owens & Minor, a distribution company that has stuck to its tradition of distributing medical/surgical supplies to acute care facilities, resisting the moves taken by rivals to integrate medical/surgical with pharmaceutical distribution or to move into other market segments such as physicians and long-term care. Instead, Owens & Minor has focused inwardly, emphasizing information technology and service innovations, resulting in it being named in 2001 by *Information Week* number one among *Fortune* 500 companies that use information technology.

The defender orientation was common among healthcare providers for many decades in part because of the predominance of not-for-profit ownership forms, which tended to focus on community mission rather than on gaining advantage by moving aggressively outside of their existing markets. By the 1990s, however, many not-for-profit organizations shifted toward aggressive strategic orientations (Shortell, Morrison, and Friedman 1990). Now that the turbulence of the 1990s has passed, many appear to be reverting to conservative strategic postures, possibly even becoming defenders once again.

The *analyzer* type is in the middle of the prospector and the defender. Organizations that assume this orientation tend to balance risk taking with stability by watching the environment carefully, assessing movements of competitors, and acting in response to their observations. They are thus not likely to be first movers, although they might be immediate followers of the actions taken by their prospective rivals. As such, the analyzers might be appropriately characterized as imitators, given that they monitor and copy the successful moves of competitors. Analyzers also tend to emphasize core products and technologies and established and refined strategies while investing in new product and market development. In healthcare, analyzers likely emphasize market penetration over market expansion (movement into new markets or product lines), a preference that is fairly unique to healthcare organizations (a point discussed in Chapter 7). Also, to the extent that product development is emphasized, analyzers likely prefer complimentary, as opposed to entirely new, products or businesses.

The last type is the *reactor*, which is often adaptive but not necessarily consistent or effective in its responses to environmental stimuli. Reactors characterize organizations that either lack the manpower and skills to conduct careful strategic analyses or are culturally or institutionally constrained in their strategic maneuverability (the latter is a common problem for healthcare organizations). Because their options and capabilities are limited, reactors tend to respond to threats rather than enact their strategic futures. Reactor organizations are thus expected to be relatively unstable financially; unsteady in charting coherent strategic courses; and, in general, unclear about their overall missions and directions. To the extent that this orientation is attributed to internal organizational factors, it can be modifiable. But if it is caused by external constraints, such as permanent budgetary restrictions or poor locations, this orientation might not be so readily altered.

Freestanding "downtown" or public hospitals come to mind as possible organizations that tend toward the reactor orientation. The freestanding, central-city hospital, if it is located in the heart of a large market, typically faces large, highly powerful, even dominating community systems as competitors. Community systems often have the capital and organizational capabilities to maneuver far more rapidly and effectively than is possible, say, for public hospitals, which are often constrained by approved budgets and legal restrictions. Therefore, such competitors either flail about in search of a workable strategy or are forced to change dramatically their missions and strategies, which they are greatly restrained from doing. For the change in mission and strategies to occur, these organizations can restructure themselves to enable them to function as private, independent entities. In fact, this is what Shands, a Gainesville, Florida–based academic medical center, did in 1979 when it changed from a state institution to a private hospital company. As a result of the change, Shands has grown rapidly, acquiring facilities in nearby Jacksonville and the surrounding nonurban area. Shands's strategic development has thus far outstripped many of the remaining state-owned academic medical centers, few of which have been able to make the legal and strategic adjustments accomplished by Shands. In effect, Shands has shifted from an enforced reactor orientation to one that is considerably more assertive.

More radically, public organizations can allow themselves to be acquired by, say a national for-profit chain, which is a move that many nonurban public hospitals have taken as a strategy for survival. Another option is to become a specialty or niche provider or move out of the healthcare business altogether. For example, in the mid-1960s, as Medicare and Medicaid reduced the need for many charity hospitals, Sheltering Arms Hospital, a charity hospital in Richmond, Virginia, moved to another site and became a rehabilitation hospital; it is now thriving in the Richmond area. Many reactor organizations, however, are unable to pull off such shifts in structure and overall strategic orientation.

The Miles and Snow typology in some ways applies to the shifts in strategic orientation that have occurred over the last few decades. The 1960s through the 1980s, for example, might be characterized as defender decades, in which market threat was limited and dramatic strategic moves were few. The 1990s can be seen as the prospector decade, in which much strategic maneuvering took place. The current decade, with its more cautious but determined strategic orientation, might be viewed as the decade of the analyzer. Industries go through periods and cycles in their general action orientations. The key is not to be in sync with the mood of the time but to be able to look beyond the accepted generalizations of the moment and make rational strategic decisions.

ORGANIZATIONAL CULTURE AND CAPABILITIES

Montgomery (1988) suggested that the advantages of taking timely actions depend directly on the resources and capabilities of an organization, as well as on conditions in the external environment. An organization that possesses skills in new product development, for example, might be better equipped to engage in aggressive strategic maneuvering. By contrast, organizations that are not as strong in these areas but are better, say, at marketing or delivering services might be better off waiting and following (imitating) the actions taken by market leaders. Put another way, organizations that enter into periods of rapid and significant market development might need to change not only their leadership but also their organizational structures and cultures to be capable of responding effectively (Leontiades 1980).

A good example of a relationship between internal capabilities and culture and strategic orientations can be found in the tobacco industry. In his study of the strategic orientations of tobacco manufacturers, Robert Miles (1982; not the same as the author of the Miles and Snow typology) classifies each of the leading companies using the Miles and Snow typology. Phillip Morris, for example, because of its consistent pattern of innovation and early movement (examples of which are flip-top boxes, filters, international market expansion), is categorized as a prospector. R. J. Reynolds is labeled an analyzer because it tended to follow the lead of Philip Morris and others in the industry. American Brands is a defender and, according to Miles (1982) and Ligget & Myers, is a reactor. One of Miles's important findings is that these companies tended to retain their particular strategic orientations over time. He suggests that this constant orientation can be attributed to the key roles that those companies' cultures played in establishing their distinctive strategic orientations. The culture, in other words, dictated the degree to which these companies were willing to take risks or, in effect, to be early movers.

Shortell's Comfort Zones

In an interesting contrast, Shortell, Morrison, and Friedman (1990) found that many hospitals did shift their strategic orientations over time. When they did, these hospitals tended toward orientations that were not too different from the ones they previously assumed. This suggests that the changes in orientations were done within the hospitals' *comfort zones* or only marginally. Shortell, Morrison, and Friedman's findings are actually consistent with those reported by Miles, confirming the critical role that culture plays in shaping (and constraining) how organizations respond to external threats.

We illustrate the comfort zones in Figure 5.4. As illustrated in the figure, prospectors are likely to shift to the analyzer orientation rather than to the defender, which would be a more drastic move. The reverse is true

Figure 5.4. Comfort Zones Within the Pace Source of Advantage

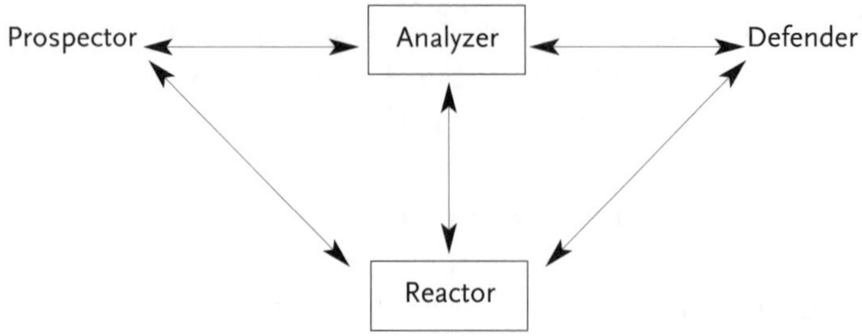

Source: Strategic Choices for America's Hospitals: Managing Change in Turbulent Times. by S. M. Shortell, E. M. Morrison, and B. Friedman. San Francisco: Jossey-Bass. Copyright © 1990. This material is used by permission of John Wiley & Sons, Inc.

for the defenders. Analyzers, being in the middle of the strategic orientations (in terms of willingness to take risks), can change to being either prospectors or defenders. Reactors, however, can switch to any of the three types depending on the degree of aggressiveness with which they had been pursuing strategy in the first place.

The comfort zone concept reinforces the role of cultural congruity in an organization's approach to strategy. Organizations, in other words, are relatively unlikely to make major shifts in orientation without first undergoing major changes in culture, management, and structure.

CONCLUSION

Remaining cautious obviously offers security, but taking bold actions offers some psychic satisfaction. Which of the two is the better posture often can only be judged once the evidence comes in. Many highly visible examples of successful strategic initiatives can be found, but, unfortunately, many relics of failed actions taken by early movers also exist. This is as true in healthcare as in any other industry. No formula for action fits every situation.

Peters and Waterman's first of eight principles of excellence—a bias for action—can be taken as an expressed preference for early or first movement. Alternatively, it can be seen as a call for readiness should action be needed. Of course, costs are associated with maintaining strategic readiness—that is, investments must be made in learning, staff development, data acquisition, leadership training, and so forth. But the costs of premature strategic movements or ill-advised caution can be far greater.

The drivers of strategy are rarely fully predictable. In fact, the action may already be too late as soon as the need for action is recognized; thus, a strategic orientation toward learning and analysis is a safe prescription. Besides, readiness comes with other benefits. An organization engaged in strategic analysis is likely to find many opportunities for refinement along the way.

REFERENCES

Ansoff, I. 1977. "Managing Surprise and Discontinuity: Strategic Response to Weak Signals." In *Strategy + Structure = Performance: The Strategic Planning Imperative*, edited by H. B. Thorelli, 53-82. Bloomington, IN: Indiana University Press.

Chakravarthy, B. S. 1982. "Adaptation: A Promising Metaphor for Strategic Management." *Academy of Management Review* 7 (3): 35–44.

D'Aveni, R. A. 1994. *Hypercompetition: Managing the Dynamics of Strategic Maneuvering*. New York: The Free Press.

Harrigan, K. 1985. *Strategic Flexibility: A Management Guide for Changing Times*. Lexington, MA: Lexington Books.

Henderson, B. D. 1979. *On Corporate Strategy*. Cambridge, MA: Abt Books.

Jones, A. 1987. *The Art of War in the Western World*. New York: Oxford University Press.

Leontiades, M. 1980. *Strategies for Diversification and Change*. Boston: Little Brown and Co.

Lieberman, M. B., and D. B. Montgomery. 1998. "First-Mover (Dis)Advantages: Retrospective and Link with the Resource-Based View." *Strategic Management Journal* 19: 1111–125.

MacMillan, I. C. 1984. "Seizing Competitive Initiative." In *Competitive Strategic Management*, edited by R. Lamb, 272–96. Englewood Cliffs, NJ: Prentice-Hall.

Miles, R. E., and C. C. Snow. 1978. *Organizational Strategy, Structure, and Process*. New York: McGraw-Hill.

Miles R. 1982. *Coffin Nails and Corporate Strategies*. Englewood Cliffs, NJ: Prentice-Hall.

Mintzberg, H. 1978. "Patterns in Strategy Formation." *Management Science* 24 (9): 934–48.

Montgomery, C. A. 1988. "Introduction to the Special Issue on Research in the Content of Strategy." *Strategic Management Journal* 9: 3–8.

Peters, T., and R. Waterman. 1982. *In Search of Excellence*. New York: Harper & Row.

Porter, M. 1980. *Competitive Strategy*. New York: The Free Press.

―――. 1985. *Competitive Advantage: Creating and Sustaining Superior Performance*. New York: The Free Press.

Rothschild, W. E. 1984. "Surprise and the Competitive Advantage." *The Journal of Business Strategy* 4 (3): 10–18.

Shortell, S. M., E. M. Morrison, and B. Friedman. 1990. *Strategic Choices for America's Hospitals: Managing Change in Turbulent Times*. San Francisco: Jossey-Bass.

Waterman, R., Jr., T. Peters, and J. R. Phillips. 1980. "Structure Is Not Organisation." *Business Horizons* 23 (3): 14–26.

Yoffie, D. B., and M. Kwak. 2001. *Judo Strategy: Turning Your Competitors' Strength to Your Advantage*. Boston: Harvard Business School Press.

Chapter 6

Position, Potential, and Performance Strategies

Therefore there are five factors in anticipating which side will win.... The side that knows when to fight and when not to.... The side that understands how to deal with numerical superiority and inferiority.... The side that has superiors and subordinates united in purpose.... The side that fields a fully prepared army against one that is not.... The side on which the commander is able and the ruler does not interfere....

—*Sun-Tzu (Carr 2000, 80)*

IN THIS CHAPTER, we explore three additional sources of advantage—position, potential, and performance—that have been at the center of the debate about the sources of competitive advantage. Despite the market structure view that favors positioning and the resource-based view that favors potential and performance, strategy analysts must not take sides but consider any and all sources that advance and help to sustain advantage. In our discussion of position strategies, we revisit Porter's argument that there exist two primary "generic" positions: low cost and high differentiation; the applicability of these two to healthcare organizations will be discussed. Provider organizations, especially, are likely to pursue not just one or the other position but more than one at a time (called "dual advantages").

In discussing potential strategies, which have to do with attaining distinctive capabilities or resources, we focus on sustaining distinctiveness in the face of competitor efforts to duplicate those advantages. Two primary threats to distinctiveness—imitation and substitution—are explored. Performance strategies involve strategy monitoring and control, which are examined in this chapter from strategic planning and value chain perspectives.

POSITION

In defending his arguments about competitive advantage, Porter (1996, 63) suggests that the successes and failures of Japanese competition illustrate the central role positioning plays in competitive strategy. He posits that one reason Japanese competitors might have lost some of their competitive punch is that they have paid too much attention to operational efficiencies (which he considers a management concern) and given too little emphasis to positioning (which he believes is the central focus of strategy). One can challenge the validity of Porter's points in at least two respects. First, many Japanese companies have, in fact, been very successful in carving out strong positions in their markets; see for example the high-quality positions (let alone low-price positions in a number of cases) attained by such Japanese companies as Lexus, Infinity, Sony, and Toshiba. Second, Porter is wrong in relegating operational efficiencies and performance to mere management concerns. In some cases, they can be seen as management concerns and in others as being essential for generating competitive advantage. However, he is right in emphasizing the strategic importance of positioning.

For too long, *positioning* has languished in the field of marketing and been given insufficient attention in the field of strategy. As a tool of marketing, positioning applies mostly to projecting value to consumers for individual products and services. At the strategic level, it applies to organizations as a whole. As such, it deals with the collective efforts by complex organizations to project and sustain value in the eyes of their consumers and to convert this value into competitive advantage.

Beyond the Generic Strategies

Porter also makes the case that organizations, if they hope to be successful strategically, should pursue one of three *generic strategies* or positions. Technically, there are only two generic positions; the third is just a narrowed version of the other two:

- Low cost
- High differentiation
- Focus (pursue customer niches with either low-cost or high-differentiation strategies)

Differentiation embodies a great variety of dimensions by which organizations distinguish themselves in the marketplace. In the hospital sector, for example, competitors differentiate themselves by quality, location, level of specialization, service orientation, convenience, technical competency, religious affiliation, ownership type, system model, and so on.

By modifying positions with the term "generic," Porter was arguing that organizations were best off if they pursued one or the other of the two major alternatives, but not both. Is he right about this? Should they not also pursue dual advantages (Ghemawat 2000, 56), which simultaneously emphasize high differentiation and low cost? What about the viability of pursuing a middle position—somewhere in between the two generic positions? The primary argument against such hybrid positions is that each of the two extreme positions requires different business models. The kinds of management approaches, leadership, organizational structures, and cultures required to achieve low-cost positions differ greatly from those required to achieve positions of high differentiation. Optimality considerations thus suggest that one or the other position must be taken, not both.

Food Lion (see Chapter 1) provides a good example of a company that focuses on a single generic position: low cost. The company achieves savings through the use of highly trained management teams, standard formats in store and warehouse design and management, close coordination with suppliers, technological advances in the pursuit of energy efficiencies (e.g., computerized control of freezers), and many other cost-saving strategies. Its intended low-cost position is clearly expressed in the tag line that often accompanies the company logo: "Saving you time and money is our business. What you do with the savings is yours." It would be difficult for Food Lion to sustain a position of low cost while also being positioned as a highly differentiated supermarket chain. To also emphasize product diversity, quality, and customer service would require investments in additional management and system development, which, if done, could preclude Food Lion from sustaining its low-cost position. This is Porter's point: low-cost and high-differentiation positions are incompatible with one another.

Dual Advantages

The idea that organizations should pursue one or the other generic position is reasonable, but there is no reason an organization with a low-cost position should not also seek additional advantage by strengthening its position—say, in the area of quality; the same is true for high-differentiated organizations. In fact, Food Lion, although not positioned as a high-quality supermarket chain, is fully aware that quality is important in the food business. Thus, the company sometimes places this additional statement alongside its logo: "The company maintains its low price leadership and quality assurance." By pursuing low costs while seeking to shore up its quality position, Food Lion increases the chances that it will gain some advantage over other low-cost rivals, marginally erode the markets of high-differentiated competitors, and defend against price attacks by higher-quality-positioned competitors. This point was made by Ghemawat in assessing McDonalds, a low-cost positioned company. McDonalds, he observed, has somewhat distinguished itself by carving out a stronger quality position relative to its low-cost rivals. Having achieved a slight advantage in quality, McDonalds has been able to charge a small premium over the prices of competitors.

In the hospital sector, the *dual advantages* approach is fairly common. Many community hospitals selectively invest in advanced clinical technologies and manpower. This allows them to maintain a moderate-cost position (as might be expected of a typical community provider) and at the same time claim a differentiated position in those selected areas where they compete directly with high-cost, high-quality referral rivals and academic medical centers. More importantly, these community hospitals seek to extend the quality image or position they achieved in one particular area to their entire enterprise. CJW Medical Center, a merged entity between two HCA hospitals in Richmond, Virginia, is an example of a local competitor that has taken exactly this tack. As a community hospital system, CJW invested heavily in cardiac care. Its apparent target was the historically strong high-quality and high-technology rival—the VCU Health System, a prestigious academic medical center also located in Richmond. On its web site, CJW claims that it is the number one heart hospital, not just in Richmond but in the entire state of Virginia. With this pronouncement, CJW is claiming a quality advantage over VCU as well as over other major systems in the state, such as the University of Virginia Health System in nearby Charlottesville and the Inova Health System in northern Virginia. Through careful marketing, CJW seeks to extend the reputation it gained in the cardiac area to the whole of its activities, thereby enhancing the position of the hospital overall. And it does this through selective investment in a few specialty areas.

The above examples suggest that multiple battles are ongoing in the positioning arena. One is between rivals within a particular position. Another is between organizations in opposing positions, such as between high quality and low cost. And another is between organizations that are differently differentiated, as between one that has a religious base and one that is community oriented. In all these battles, the key strategy is not just to strengthen a particular position but, as Ghemawat (2000, 57) says, to "drive the largest possible wedge between costs and differentiation" or between an organization's established (or intended) position and a competitor's position. The pursuit of dual or multiple advantages is clearly a viable approach for doing this. This approach is especially practical in the healthcare industry, where market pressures on cost, quality, service, and other dimensions of care are strong.

Middle Position

Another assumption based on the concept of generic strategies is that a *middle position* (between low cost and high differentiation) is not at all viable. This assumption is contradicted by the many supermarket, apparel, hardware, and other companies that do very well in middle positions; they offer middle-range quality products at middle-range prices. In fact, the middle might be the dominant and strongest position for many consumer product markets. In many such instances, the two generic extremes actually tend to be niche rather than dominating positions.

In the hospital sector, both middle- and high-differentiation positions are clearly among the most desirable. In fact, the majority of the community acute care general hospitals fall in the middle area; the smaller number of teaching, referral, and specialty hospitals occupy high-differentiation positions (e.g., the Shriners Hospitals for Children–Houston Unit or The University of Texas M. D. Anderson Cancer Center, both of which are located in the Texas Medical Center in Houston, Texas).

Low-Cost Position

Is the low-cost, low-differentiation position viable for healthcare providers? (Technically, this position refers to low price because it is the "price," not the "cost" that the consumer sees.) The managed care environment in the 1990s placed a high premium on low costs and prices. This preference manifested itself more in direct negotiations between managed care companies and provider systems than in the market choices made by the users of services. Moreover, negotiations with the managed care companies tended to become power struggles, in which those possessing the greatest leverage (because of size and, in the case of providers, control over critical market areas for which the managed care companies needed to provide coverage) fared better. As is widely recognized, most managed care plans include most of the local providers in their networks, regardless of their relative costs. Thus, even as a strategy to gain managed care contracts, the low-cost position provides no real advantage among local providers.

One might argue that for-profit suburban hospitals occupy low-cost, low-differentiation positions. Small, suburban, for-profit hospitals are often considered low on the service diversity and quality spectrum; however, whether or not they are low cost, these hospitals tend not to be low priced. In fact, research supports the conclusion that for-profit and not-for-profit hospitals differ little on costs, but for profits tend to be higher priced (Clement et al. 1997).

In general, low-cost positions (as perceived by the users of health services) are not desirable in the provider sector. Low costs are too easily associated with low quality, which is obviously not a very sensible position to assume in an industry that provides services to the sick and dying. This, of course, does not mean that there is no strategic advantage to being low cost; in fact, being a low-cost provider offers such competitors important flexibility in difficult economic times. For example, it can provide a much-needed cushion if compromise is required in negotiations with managed care companies, or it can free up scarce resources to support other strategic objectives. In any case, healthcare providers are generally averse to being positioned as low cost, unless they can convince the consuming public that they are high quality as well. A low-cost position in the provider sector works if a dual-advantage approach is pursued and if combined with high quality.

High-Quality Position

Ironically, despite the unmistakable importance of quality in healthcare, not as many competitors as expected have been able to establish distinctively high quality positions. In general, the public has great difficulty judging quality differences and making choices among providers based on such differences; also, it tends to assume that most providers provide good quality care. The fact that physicians practice within fragmented market structures makes it highly difficult for consumers to distinguish positions on quality. On the acute care side, patients encounter hospitals infrequently and sporadically and thus rarely have the opportunity to compare quality or services across hospitals (even if they were capable of doing so, and they probably are not). The academic medical centers and referral hospitals are important exceptions because of the distinctive roles they play in providing complex, tertiary, and quaternary services. But even they have not always established uncontested positions on quality. Many of these sophisticated provider systems also serve as healthcare safety nets for the poor and disadvantaged, especially if they are public institutions. In addition, many occupy undesirable downtown locations. All of these and other characteristics complicate their attempts to establish and sustain undisputed high-quality positions. The expansion of the Minnesota-based Mayo Clinic into Arizona and Florida and The Cleveland Clinic into Florida is clearly based on assumptions that these systems enjoy high-quality positions, not just locally but nationally and even internationally. In the future, it will be interesting to see if other similarly distinguished systems will be able to capitalize on their distinctive reputations as have these two nationally recognized systems.

Many integrated systems have been able to extend to their local community hospitals and other healthcare business the positions attained by their highly visible and respected hub facilities (see discussion of hub-spoke configurations in Chapter 8). These systems, in effect, combine the benefits of organizational mass and market power with the advantages of high-quality positioning. By joining community facilities with referral centers, these integrated systems might also be able to rationalize the distribution of services and thus enhance their ability to attain lower-cost positions than otherwise might be possible. To the extent that such strategies are successful in the future, high-quality positioning could become very difficult to beat.

Dynamics of Positioning

At any time, competitors tend to be spread out across the positioning dimensions of cost and differentiation. With continued competition, they are likely to shift their positions over time, especially if their rivals have recently attained, or are expected to try to attain, positions that are superior to their own. For reasons already discussed, most organizations will gravitate toward one generic position but can, at any time, find themselves at some unintended point within the two-dimensional plane of generic extremes.

Figure 6.1 illustrates the range of positions that are generally available to competitors. In the figure, three levels for each of the two positions are identified—high, medium, and low; the figure can be expanded to many more levels and even can be converted into a continuous scale. Porter's generic positions are located along the diagonal. Contrary to Porter's argument, the middle position is also defined as a generic position, which fits well with the strategies pursued by healthcare providers. The generic

Figure 6.1. Range and Migration of Positions

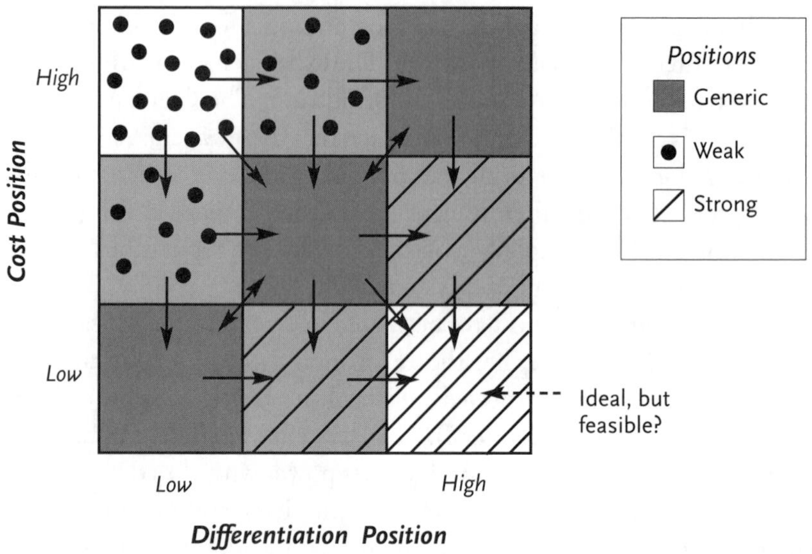

positions include low cost/low differentiation, moderate cost/moderate differentiation (middle position), and high cost/high differentiation.

Over time, organizations will shift among the generic positions; for example, low-cost or high-differentiation companies might move toward the center or center-positioned companies might move to the extremes. In reality, *mobility barriers* or feasibility restraints that inhibit major strategic shifts (see Chapter 4) are likely to prevent major movements between widely diverse strategic positions. Marginal shifts in position are more likely, which are indicated in the figure by the arrows. Clearly, positions in the upper left side of the cube (the dotted cells) are weak relative to the other strategies. Either moderate cost/low differentiation or high cost/moderate differentiation will always trump high cost/low differentiation (all other things being equal). Thus, competitors in those dotted areas are expected to attempt to move toward any of the three generic positions. A number of hospitals actually occupy high cost/low differentiation positions (the dark dotted cell), which in most markets are not viable at all. These include, in particular, many public hospitals (e.g., the John H. Stroger Hospital of Cook County in Chicago) that serve segmented populations (e.g., low income, minority, trauma) with adequate quality and at relatively low levels of efficiency. Perhaps in

Porter's terms, these hospital can be classified as pursuing a focus or niched position.

Positions that fall in the striped zone, by contrast, are superior to the supposed generic positions (gray zones). Low cost/moderate differentiation, for example, should trump low cost/low differentiation. In effect, the middle generic (gray) and the striped zone positions are where competitors have captured dual advantages. In the end, all positions tend to gravitate toward the lower right corner—low cost/high differentiation, which is the optimal strategic position, although a difficult one to attain and sustain.

In a competitive and turbulent environment (one in which information and clinical technologies are changing rapidly), the requirements for occupying one or another position will change. An organization that is initially located in a low cost/low differentiation position might be surprised to find that its location shifted into the weak zone at some point in the future. This can happen if the organization's rivals worked hard to lower its costs or improve its ability to differentiate itself. Therefore, organizations need to be vigilant about sustaining established positions and, in competitive market environments, work to improve those positions. Positioning threats can come from similarly positioned rivals; from rivals located in other, stronger positions (gray and striped zones); or from rivals that need to improve on weak positions (dotted zones).

Protected Position

Competitors can find shelter from ongoing position competition. For example, some competitors are so highly differentiated or enjoy such unassailable cost advantages that the resulting mobility barriers shield them from any significant position competition. Many of the large, high-reputation academic and referral centers have long been protected from competition because of the historically technologically advanced, high-quality, research-based care they provide. Other organizations have found protection in geographic niches. Location has always been a highly important differentiator and a strong position protector. Many acute care providers operate within relatively uncontested geographic niches, either in suburban or in nonurban areas. Relatively speaking, these providers are much less likely to have to compete actively for position, or, for that matter, to compete aggressively using other sources of advantage. Geographic protection, however, does not generally extend to the competitors that operate in the center of large urban markets. Nearly every large market has at least two, and sometimes many more, major hospital competitors that are tightly clustered within those areas. Lacking geographic buffering, these competitors are likely engaged in direct position competition. Also, they are likely to be involved in other forms of strategic maneuvering, especially that of merging with nearby rivals and acquiring other hospitals in their markets.

Many of the so-called protected positions are losing some of their protected distinctiveness. Community and specialty hospitals are competing in selected areas with academic and referral centers. Urban hospitals are reaching out to the markets of historically protected nonurban providers, and many suburban hospitals now are experiencing competition from the outpatient surgery centers and clinics that are established in their areas by their downtown rivals. Overall, with technological change and market evolution, most healthcare providers need to watch out for position competition, even in areas that for decades were considered safe.

POTENTIAL

Potential refers to the distinctive internal resources and capabilities that might give advantage to an organization in the design and implementation of its strategies. Table 6.1 categorizes the important internal resources that produce competitive advantage by whether they are tangible and intangible.

Most of these resources are important in healthcare. Many healthcare organizations, for example, enjoy highly capable professional staffs who have strong reputations for providing quality. Others gain advantage from their memberships in multihospital systems or purchasing alliances, and others achieve it by investing in advanced information systems and modern and attractive physical facilities. The key to assessing all such resources is to determine which ones produce competitive advantage and whether their strategic potential can be sustained.

Sustainability

Resources have to be both strategically important and sustainable. The first is somewhat easier to assess because value tends to be either self-evident or relatively easy to figure out. Sustainability, on the other hand, is much more subtle and difficult to ascertain. This is because conclusions about sustainability derive from analyses of competitor behaviors, intentions, and capabilities, which are not so readily identifiable. Good market intelligence and analysis are essential in this case.

Table 6.1. Resources and Capabilities of an Organization

Tangible (Resources)
- Financial (structure, cash flow, capital base, profitability)
- Physical plant, property (condition, age, modernity)
- Service capacity/mix
- Organization structure (tightness, centralization)
- Partnerships, alliances
- Systems (information systems, control systems, clinical integration, etc.)
- Technology
- Clinical and/or administrative manpower
- Location

Intangible (Capabilities)
- Experience
- Reputation
- Culture
- Specialized skills and knowledge (e.g., "system" skills, clinical, management)
- Communication, analytic, interactive skills
- Distinctive organizational "routines"
- Motivation
- Innovativeness

Threats to sustainability come in two forms—imitation and substitution (Ghemawat 2000). *Imitation* has to do with whether rivals are able or willing to duplicate a competitor's sources of competitive advantage. *Substitution* involves an indirect threat from rivals that put forward substitute products or adopt alternative business models. Our primary interest is in the combinations of resources and capabilities that in their totality produce significantly different business models. (See discussion on product substitution in Chapter 4.)

Imitation

Direct imitation is perhaps the most common and powerful way for a competitor to erode the advantages of rivals. The essence of market competition in this area is when organizations learn from one another and copy each other's activities. The challenge facing any competitor, therefore, is to build advantages that cannot easily be duplicated by rivals. Rumelt (1987) called this the building of "isolating mechanisms," a term he borrowed from the field of ecology. These mechanisms prevent rivals from gaining access to the kinds of resources on which an organization bases its advantage. Others have called these "barriers to imitation" (Reed and DeFillippi 1990), a term we prefer because it is consistent with other barriers considered in the field of strategy, such as entry, exit, and mobility. Mobility barriers (see Chapter 4) are actually similar to imitation barriers, except that the former apply broadly to the constraints that limit members of given strategic groups from imitating or adopting the business models pursued by members of other strategic groups. *Imitation barriers*, by contrast, arise at a somewhat lower unit of analysis. They refer to the constraints that rivals face as they seek to copy the capabilities of direct competitors.

Table 6.2 lists some important barriers to imitation, which can be grouped into four categories—transparency, access, competitive, and institutional. *Transparency barriers* include factors that prevent rivals from either seeing or understanding the sources of a competitor's advantage. With transparency barriers, a large provider system's evolved, unique approaches to monitoring performance at all levels cannot be observed or, if observed, cannot be understood by its rivals. *Access barriers* include factors that stop rivals from accessing the distinctive resources of given competitors, even if such resources were observable. Those resources might be either rare or not readily movable across organizations or space. For example, access barriers increase if a competitor is successful in locking in its distinctive resources (say, by paying high salaries or obtaining a patent), thereby making it difficult for rivals to bid the resources away. Again, the academic medical centers provide a good example of the role access barriers can play in healthcare. Their distinctive educational and research functions have long provided a strong barrier that prevents community hospitals from drawing away their highly specialized and often prestigious academic faculty. However, as already discussed, such barriers have fallen in the face of technological change and increases in the size and resource bases of many community rivals.

Competitive barriers include a wide variety of factors, ranging from scale economies to first-mover advantages and learning. These factors increase the costs and risks associated with imitative moves by rivals. For example, in the 1990s, many hospital systems were able to build up sufficient organizational mass and market power for them to credibly threaten retaliation if, say, systems located in nearby markets were to contemplate entering their markets.

Table 6.2. Barriers to Imitation

Transparency
- Proprietary knowledge
- Strategic complexity, system interconnectedness

Access
- Rarity
- Immobility (geographically, organizationally)

Competitive
- Threats of retaliation
- Economies of scale, scope
- Distinctive positions (e.g., unique locations, reputations)
- Learning, developmental history, time lags
- Special arrangements (contracts, relationships, networks, partnerships)

Institutional
- Legal/regulatory (certificate of need, trademarks, patents, tax status)
- Sociocultural, religious, moral
- Professional

Sources: Concepts from Barney, J. 1991. "Firm Resources and Sustained Competitve Advantage." *Journal of Management* 17 (1): 99–120; Barney, J. 1996. "The Resource-Based Theory of the Form." *Organizational Service* 7 (5): 469; Bourgeois, L., I. Duhaime, and J. Stimpert. 1999. *Strategic Management: Concepts for Managers*, 2nd ed. Fort Worth, TX: Dryden Press; Ghemawat, P. 2000. *Strategy and the Business Landscape: Core Concepts*. Upper Saddle River, NJ: Prentice Hall; Grant, R. 1998. "The Resource-Based Theory of Competitive Advantage: Implications for Strategy Formulation." In *The Strategy Reader*, edited by S. Segal Horn, 179–99. Malden, MA: Blackwell; Rumelt, R. P. 1987. "Theory, Strategy, and Entrepreneurship." In *The Competitive Challenge: Strategies for Industrial Innovation and Renewal*, edited by D. J. Teese, 136–52. Cambridge, MA: Ballinger.

Finally, *institutional barriers* can slow imitation; such barriers include all of the restraints on strategic action that reside within the legal, regulatory, religious, professional, and other institutions, all of which greatly influence strategy in the healthcare industry. Catholic hospital systems, for example, because of a variety of religious and hierarchical considerations (institutional constraints), are highly restricted in the kinds of hospitals they might seek to acquire. This has limited Catholic systems' ability to imitate the market-dominating moves of aggressive, not religiously affiliated, not-for-profit competitors.

Substitution

In the 1990s, threats of alternative business models became far more prevalent than in prior decades. Many new system arrangements or distinct corporate/business unit configurations proliferated in that decade, not only in the provider sector but in managed care as well. These new arrangements introduced considerably more strategic complexity and risk into healthcare markets.

Substitution presents a very different competitive threat to that of imitation. Substitute models often come out of left field, so to speak, and they often involve significant innovations (Christensen 1997), which means the emerging models are sometimes not recognizable until they emerge and succeed. Substitute models can make obsolete the technologies and strategies of established business models. On the other hand, they also can fail to mount a viable challenge because competitors that pursue them often enter the markets very high up on the learning curve and filled with uncertainties, which lead them to significant risks.

The strategic challenge for substitution is to anticipate the emerging threats. Table 6.3 identifies two primary reasons that substitutes can pose a serious threat to competitors: (1) failure to observe the substitution threat and (2) once observed, failure to respond in a timely manner. The latter has been a serious problem in the provider sector and is caused by many factors.

Strategic Responses to Substitution

Ghemawat (2000) identifies a number of strategic responses for competitors in the face of concrete threats from substitution:

- Fight
- Switch
- Recombine (hybrid)
- Straddle (do both)
- Harvest

The first (fight) can be adopted as a strategy if a competitor is fairly sure that the new business model is vulnerable and can be resisted. The second (switch) suggests that a competitor capitulates and adopts the new model, which the competitor perceives to be superior to its own; this, obviously, is not an easy thing to do, given well-recognized institutional and mobility barriers. The third (recombine) involves the formulation of an

Table 6.3. Reasons for Failed Responses to Rival Substitution Threats

Failure to observe the substitution threat
- Environmental changes not well understood (e.g., shifts in sociodemographics, consumer preferences)
- Involves technological innovations
- Involves business model innovations

Failure to respond in a timely manner, due to
- Organizational inertia (e.g., lack of environmental scanning, internal politics; institutional constraints)
- Strategic overconfidence (e.g., overreliance on established sources of competitve advantage; assumptions about the markets)

Sources: Concepts from Christensen, C. M. 1997. *The Innovator's Dilemma: When New Technologies Cause Great Firms to Fail.* Boston: Harvard Business School Press; Ghemawat, P. 2000. *Strategy and the Business Landscape: Core Concepts.* Upper Saddle River, NJ: Prentice Hall.

entirely new business model that combines the perceived strengths of the incumbent organization with those of the substitute. Allina, a major player in Minneapolis, Minnesota, is a good example of an organization that attempted a hybrid strategy as a way to compete with the group model form of HMO. In 1993, Allina conjoined two companies—a hospital company (HealthSpan) and a managed care company (Medica)—into a vertically integrated delivery system. This merger, which was considered a model for many hospital systems in the 1990s, attempted to capture the advantages of the group model HMO without the hospital company giving up control. The end result, as we now know, is that in 2001 the two companies came apart; this is not an unexpected outcome, given the difficulties inherent in holding together hybrid models.

The fourth (straddle) is a variation of the hybrid response. The latter, however, is more integrative, whereas the straddle model is likely to operate the combined businesses relatively independently. For example, a local hospital system threatened by, say, MedCath, a cardiac specialty company that owns or operates 13 heart hospitals as well as catheterization laboratories and other heart-related facilities, might reconfigure its cardiac capacity by building and operating separately its own highly distinctive cardiac hospital as well as a string of ambulatory heart centers. The hospital thus creates two loosely connected, but jointly owned, businesses as opposed to reconfiguring the two entities into a new business form (the Allina strategy).

The fifth (harvest) is to succumb to the superiority of the substitute model and engage in an end-stage harvest strategy. An example of this response is when a group model HMO, confronted with severe competition from the evolving independent practice association, preferred provider organization, point-of-service organization, and other managed care models, drains its investment in the unprofitable model and eventually sells out to the other managed care companies (as Kaiser Permanente did when it moved out of the Texas market).

PERFORMANCE

Performance as a source of competitive advantage draws us directly into the administrative realm and, in so doing, opens the door to nearly every element of management and control. For our purposes, we focus only on administrative activities that are directly relevant to the implementation of strategy, specifically as a source of competitive advantage. The difficulty with viewing performance this way is that performance does not contribute directly to competitive advantage, such as might the achievement of a dominant market share. Rather, as illustrated in Figure 6.2, performance contributes indirectly by enhancing the effectiveness with which the other sources foster advantage.

Nevertheless, the indirect role played by performance does not diminish its importance as a contributor to competitive advantage. Recall the old adage (attributed to Benjamin Franklin) that linked the loss of a horseshoe nail to the loss of a war, which reminds us of just how important attention to detail and process can be to the success of a strategy. It also reminds us of how easily the more dramatic contributors to competitive advantage (e.g., building market power, positioning) can overshadow the more mundane aspects of performance management. The literature on strategy has considered the management of performance primarily from two perspectives. The first—traditional planning view—ties performance to the monitoring and control functions within a corporate planning framework. The second—competitive advantage view—links performance directly to the achievement of specific strategic objectives.

Traditional Planning View

Decades before the 1980s, strategy had been developed within highly formal and often complex strategic planning frameworks. Despite criticisms

Figure 6.2. Contribution of Performance

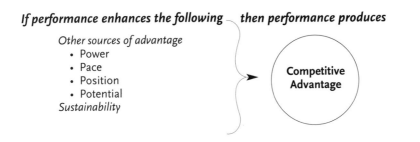

If performance enhances the following — *then performance produces*

Other sources of advantage
- Power
- Pace
- Position
- Potential

Sustainability

Competitive Advantage

(Mintzberg 1994), this framework fit fairly well the purpose to which it was applied: to enable large corporations to manage their diverse business units. This is how Lorange (1980, 18) described this approach in his book on corporate planning:

> At the corporate level the primary strategic task [is] to develop a favorable portfolio strategy for diverse business activities....The corporate level [is] concerned primarily with strategic resource flows to and from the various businesses and providing a strategy for improving the quality of the portfolio.

Thus, the role of corporate was primarily to decide on what bases resources should be distributed among its subsidiaries. To do this, corporate leaders formulated objectives that provided the guidelines by which divisional managers would identify projects they would then propose back to corporate. Corporate would assess the various proposals in the context of the objectives and changes expected in the environment. Projects would be approved and factored into the budgets that corporate would then set for the divisions. At this point, the objectives and budgets served a second purpose—to be the framework within which future performance would be monitored and evaluated. Mintzberg (1994, 78) referred to the separation between the two stages as the "great divide" in strategic planning, separating "action planning" from "performance control." The management of performance in this case served a watchdog function, informing corporate leaders of business unit progress. It also served to motivate divisional leaders to achieve the objectives established by corporate. Armed with the information gained from performance control, corporate leaders could then either adjust the objectives and budgets or

Figure 6.3. Performance as a Monitoring Function in a Traditional Strategic Planning Process

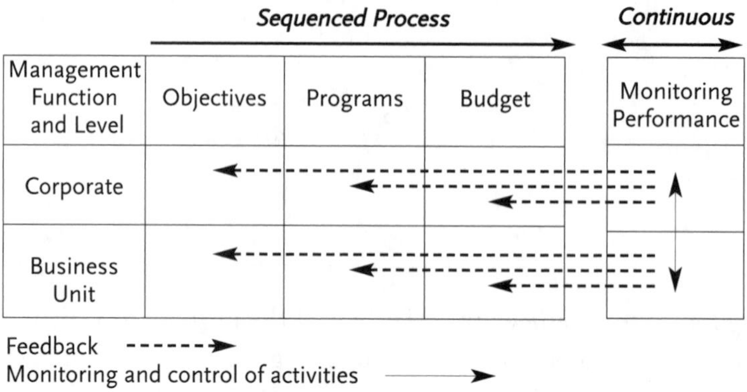

Management Function and Level	Objectives	Programs	Budget	Monitoring Performance
	Sequenced Process →			*Continuous* ←→
Corporate				
Business Unit				

Feedback - - - - - →
Monitoring and control of activities ————→

Source: CORPORATE PLANNING by Lorange, Peter ©. Reprinted by permission of Pearson Education, Inc., Upper Saddle River, NJ.

decide to withdraw their commitments to particular projects altogether.

In his book on corporate planning, Lorange (1980) provides a fairly succinct presentation of the extant thinking on this process. Figure 6.3 presents our adaptation of his view of the role corporate plays in controlling divisional performance. In the figure, which identifies four primary stages of corporate planning (objectives, programs, budget, and monitoring), the monitoring stage is highlighted, a stage that we equate to Mintzberg's performance control stage. As illustrated, this stage is both interactive, providing control along the vertical structure, and iterative, providing feedback to leadership so that objectives and budgets can be modified as needed.

Unfortunately, as Mintzberg pointed out in his extensive criticism of strategic planning, a significant detail (that is, strategy analysis) tended to be overlooked in the process of formulating strategy. Mintzberg blamed this and most other flaws on the excessive emphasis commonly placed on elaboration, quantification, and formalization in planning. The planning models often became very complex both as presented by academics and as implemented in practice. As suggested earlier, however, Mintzberg's criticisms might have missed the point. This cumbersome process was originally designed to coordinate strategies within multidivisional, portfolio business models. If applied to just those models, the process served fairly well its intended purposes. But if applied to more integrative models (see Chapter 7), the process became far too clumsy and nondirective. The strategic planning model, by design, allowed corporate to have little involvement in strategy formulation, but it focused the attention of corporate where it belonged—on financial control. Also, the model provided corporate with a framework within which it could use performance management to generate competitive advantage.

Competitive Advantage View

Obviously, the process of planning and monitoring is and should be quite different for organizations that are more integrated and in which corporate leaders are more involved in formulating strategy. In this case, performance management should be viewed as a direct contributor to advantage rather than merely as a monitoring function to be carried out hierarchically.

Porter's (1985) discussion of the *value chain* provides undoubtedly the best conceptualization of the role that performance management can play in building competitive advantage. An organization's value chain is a diagrammatic disaggregation of the activities it undertakes to produce its products and services and to carry out its strategies (Hill and Jones 1998). By assessing their value chains, organizations can identify those areas where improvements in performance can lead to more successful execution of strategy. Porter (1985, 33) explained it this way:

> Competitive advantage cannot be understood by looking at a firm as a whole. It stems from the many discrete activities a firm performs in designing, producing, marketing, delivering and supporting its product.... The value chain disaggregates a firm into its strategically relevant activities in order to understand the behavior of costs and the existing and potential sources of differentiation.

The activities in this case include any organizational processes that are believed to play an important role in producing competitive advantage. As shown in Figure 6.4, Porter distinguished between *primary activities* (those that are directly involved in the acquisition of inputs and the production and sale of products and services) and *support activities* (those that are involved specifically in the infrastructure of the organization). However configured for analysis, the purpose of conceiving of activities within a value chain is to draw attention to those processes that are within an organization's control and that, if properly managed, can make a difference in the achievement of competitive advantage. Beyond the discrete

Figure 6.4. Performance Strategy: Managing Activities in the Value Chain

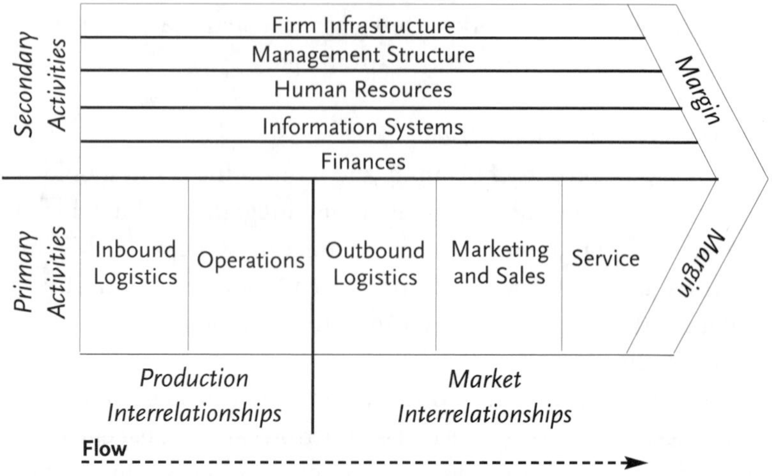

Source: Adapted with the permission of The Free Press, a Division of Simon & Schuster Adult Publishing Group, from COMPETITIVE ADVANTAGE: Creating and Sustaining Superior Performance by Michael E. Porter. Copyright © 1985, 1998 by Michael E. Porter.

activities presented in the figure, Porter (1985, 48) also suggested that organizations might need to examine the interrelationships among activities:

> Value activities are related by linkages within the value chain. Linkages are relationships between the way one value activity is performed and the cost or performance of another.... Linkages can lead to competitive advantage in two ways: optimization and coordination.

Optimization reflects the need to make tradeoffs across activities, and *coordination* is the need to ensure that interrelated activities are assessed and managed jointly.

Porter specifically applied *value chain analysis* to positioning enhancement, but it can apply to all sources of competitive advantage. An organization that seeks to move aggressively in developing new product lines or in entering new markets, for example, might find great benefit in conducting a value chain analysis. Doing so might ensure that the new ventures get off to a successful start or that rapid movement is not slowed by some unexpected breakdowns within or between key activities. The

Figure 6.5. Key to Achieving Fit (Synergies) Across Local Hospitals

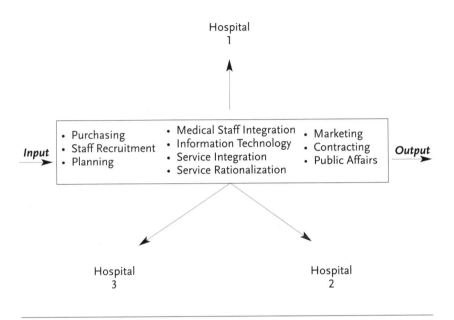

point is that one can use value chain analysis as a tool to minimize the possibility that internal management and system failures do not hamper strategic success, no matter the source of advantage.

Value Chains and Interorganizational Integration

Value chain analysis should be seen as generic to all levels and combinations of organizations because it applies well beyond single business units. It pertains most especially to multiunit organizations in which the combined entities are integrated for the purposes of maximizing advantage, such as in closely configured horizontal expansion models (see Chapter 8) or in vertical integration models (see Chapter 9). As illustrated in Figure 6.5, a combination of hospitals, especially if locally configured, can share virtually any activity, whether primary or supporting.

Porter (1996, 73) referred to the successful fitting of the individual organizational units to the whole as ensuring "organizational fit." This idea of fitting together or integrating multiple organizations is grounded in assumptions that economies will result from the integration. Such combinations themselves can be the source of competitive advantage, especially if rivals cannot easily imitate the value gained from integration. Porter said:

It is harder for a rival to match an array of interlocked activities than it is merely to imitate a particular sales-force approach, match a process technology, or replicate a set of product features. Positions built on systems of activities are far more sustainable than those built on individual activities.

In addition to fit and integration, a number of other terms have been used to identify possible advantages of interorganization combination, including complementarities, economies of scale, economies of scope, synergies, dominant logic, and corporate coherence (Prahalad and Bettis 1986; Teece et al. 1994; Milgrom and Roberts 1995; Ansoff 1965). Each of these terms refers to slightly different ways by which integration across organizational units can contribute to gains, over what might be possible if such units operated independently. Complementarities, for example, refers to the possibility that one competency or product enhances another if they are packaged together. Economies of scale refers to efficiency gains attributable to expanding the use of fixed assets. Synergies applies to nearly any gain that emanates from joint operation of multiple business units.

Despite the extensive literature devoted to the advantages of multiorganizational combinations, the evidence on synergies is mixed (Mahajan and Wind 1988). This is also true for healthcare combinations, where the evidence supporting efficiencies generated from the formation of integrated systems is very preliminary and inconclusive (McCue, Clement, and Luke 1999). Still, the strategic appeal of interorganizational combinations is very great possibly because of certain advantages to be gained from increased market and organizational power (see Chapter 7) even in the absence of efficiency or quality gains from integration. One reason that such gains are not easily realized or observed is that sharing is not cost free. Furthermore, these costs vary by what is being integrated. Shortell and colleagues (1993) identified three levels of integration within hospital-based integrated systems and pointed out that the complexity and costs of integration differ significantly across levels. As shown in Figure 6.6, difficulties in management increase when moving from mere administrative integration (across support activities) to the administrative coordination of hospitals and medical staffs (across business units) and to clinical integration (of health services for individual patients). In the 1990s, clinical integration, the most costly and complex of the three, provided a primary rationale for the aggressive attempts by many hospitals to form integrated delivery systems. Today, hospital systems, while still pursuing clinical integration, appear to

Figure 6.6. Levels of Provider Integration Within Systems

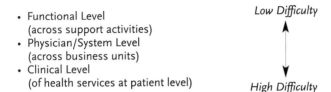

- Functional Level
  (across support activities)
- Physician/System Level
  (across business units)
- Clinical Level
  (of health services at patient level)

Low Difficulty

High Difficulty

Source: Shortell S. M., R. R. Gillies, D. Anderson, J. Mitchell, and K. Morgan. 1993. "Creating Organized Delivery Systems: The Barriers and Facilitators." *Hospital & Health Services Administration* 38 (4): 447–66.

be shifting their emphasis, at least for the moment, to the more easily captured efficiencies of administrative coordination.

The Costs of Synergies/Integration

Porter (1980) identified three categories of costs that must be balanced against the gains of sharing:

1. Costs of coordination
2. Costs of compromise
3. Costs of inflexibility

The integration of two or more hospitals in a local market, for example, certainly involves many meetings and negotiations, which consume a significant amount of time of individuals highly placed within the combined organizations. It might also involve extensive investments in information systems that would be needed for the joined organizations to standardize and enhance interorganizational communications. These are the costs of coordination. The costs of compromise might also be very great, especially for integration at the clinical level. For example, clinicians from one organization might have established clinical and administrative protocols that, with integration, might have to be modified to accommodate requirements for standardization. Finally, integration introduces inflexibility that would not be present if integration were not attempted. Joined entities needing to make rapid strategic decisions, for example, might face far more complex administrative hurdles to adaptation and change than if they functioned independently.

In sum, integration across multiple units and the management of performance for strategic advantage can be very challenging. But if successfully pursued, many additional advantages (e.g., increased market power, lower costs, improved market positions) are likely to be accomplished with greater success.

The holistic approach to value chain management might not be easily accomplished in healthcare, especially for provider organizations. This is because provider value chains are neither linear nor singular given the diversity and number of pathways through which services and patients flow within and across healthcare organizations. In acute care hospitals, for example, patients enter the system to receive highly customized care for myriad medical conditions. Even the administrative structures are very complicated because of the diversity of administrative and other functions (i.e., payment management, admissions, patient records, quality assurance, supply channel management, referral approvals) that are provided by healthcare organizations. The various clinical and administrative interorganizational relationships (such as might be established across provider and facilities in an integrated delivery system) further complicate the analysis and management of healthcare value chains. Because of such complications, some suggest that the healthcare value chain is in fact broken (Kolsky 2001). All of this suggests that value chain analysis in healthcare organizations can produce significant performance improvements, but the task of conducting such analyses is at best daunting.

CONCLUSION

This chapter addresses three very important and highly interrelated sources of competitive advantage that are especially important in healthcare: positioning, building potential advantages, and improving performance. With regard to positioning, for example, healthcare organizations might find considerable value in building strong positions of quality that are grounded in high-quality and highly distinctive (neither inimitable nor substitutable) internal resources and capabilities.

It is somewhat of a mystery that quality has not emerged as a major strategic weapon in this industry to the degree that it has, say, in the automobile or electronics industries. Certainly, quality must be highly valued by the consumers of healthcare, and, just as certainly, an organization that successfully stakes out a high-quality position (even if it comes at a high cost) should be able to gain a clear advantage. But it does not seem to work that way. Many reasons can be given for this. First, because many so-called high-quality providers often serve as safety net institutions, they might carry some stigma, diminishing the value of quality as a source of advantage. Second, patients might prefer convenience and comfort much more highly than expected; therefore, they might choose local, middle-positioned community providers over distant, possibly downtown, high-quality-positioned providers. Third, consumers might not be sufficiently aware of the quality differences. By and large, patients are unable to assess quality differences among physicians or hospitals, let alone are they generally aware of the choices available to them.

With the significant provider consolidation that has taken place, mostly among hospitals, fewer and much larger healthcare provider organizations might begin to seek out distinctive positions in the marketplace. This decade can therefore be the era in which positioning really flowers as a strategic tool for healthcare organizations. It can develop along specialty lines, with one system touting its heart hospital and the other its wellness centers, or it can emphasize the positioning of local provider collectives overall. In any case, consolidation will very likely increase the importance of positioning and associated internal capabilities as bases on which competitive advantage is attained.

REFERENCES

Ansoff, H. I. 1965. *New Corporate Strategy*. New York: McGraw-Hill.

Carr, C., ed. 2000. "Planning the Attack," translated from Sun Tzu. In *The Book of War*, 80. New York: Modern Library.

Christensen, C. M. 1997. *The Innovator's Dilemma: When New Technologies Cause Great Firms to Fail*. Boston: Harvard Business School Press.

Clement J. P., M. J. McCue, R. D. Luke, J. D. Bramble, L. F. Rossiter, Y. A. Ozcan, and C. W. Pai. 1997. "Strategic Hospital Alliances: Impact on Financial Performance." *Health Affairs* 16 (6): 193–203.

Ghemawat, P. 2000. *Strategy and the Business Landscape: Core Concepts*. Upper Saddle River, NJ: Prentice Hall.

Hill, C., and G. Jones. 1998. *Strategic Management*. Boston: Houghton Mifflin Company.

Kolsky, R. 2001. "Strategy Innovation in the Health Care Industry (or else)." *LIMBRA's MarketFacts Quarterly* 20 (4): 66–69.

Lorange, P. 1980. *Corporate Planning: An Executive Viewpoint*. Englewood Cliffs, NJ: Prentice-Hall.

Mahajan, V., and Y. Wind. 1988. "Business Synergy Does Not Always Pay Off." *Long Range Planning* 21 (1): 59–65.

McCue, M. J., J. P. Clement, and R. D. Luke. 1999. "Strategic Hospital Alliances: Do the Type and Market Structure Matter?" *Medical Care* 37 (10): 1013–22.

Milgrom, P., and J. Roberts. 1995. "Complementarities and Fit: Strategy, Structure, and Organizational Changes in Manufacturing." *Journal of Accounting and Economics* 19 (2/3): 179–208.

Mintzberg, H. 1994. *The Rise and Fall of Strategic Planning: Reconceiving Roles for Planning, Plans, Planners.* New York: The Free Press.

Porter, M. 1980. *Competitive Strategy.* New York: The Free Press.

———. 1985. *Competitive Advantage: Creating and Sustaining Superior Performance.* New York: The Free Press.

———. 1996. "What Is Strategy?" *Harvard Business Review* 74 (6): 61-78.

Prahalad, C., and R. Bettis. 1986. "The Dominant Logic: A New Linkage Between Diversity and Performance." *Strategic Management Journal* 7 (6): 485–501.

Reed, R., and R. J. DeFillippi. 1990. "Casual Ambiguity, Barriers to Imitation and Sustainable Competitive Advantage." *Academy of Management Review* 15 (1): 88–102.

Rumelt, R. P. 1987. "Theory, Strategy, and Entrepreneurship." In *The Competitive Challenge: Strategies for Industrial Innovation and Renewal*, edited by D. J. Teese, 136–52. Cambridge, MA: Ballinger.

Shortell, S. M., R. R. Gillies, D. Anderson, J. Mitchell, and K. Morgan. 1993. "Creating Organized Delivery Systems: The Barriers and Facilitators." *Hospital & Health Services Administration* 38 (4): 447–66.

Teece, D. J., R. P. Rumelt, G. Dosi, and S. G. Winter. 1994. "Understanding Corporate Coherence: Theory and Evidence." *Journal of Economic Behavior and Organization* 23 (1): 1–30.

Chapter 7

Power Strategies

The best strategy is always to be very strong, first of all generally, then at the decisive point.... [T]here is no more imperative and no simpler law for strategy than to keep the forces concentrated.

—*Clausewitz (2000, 427)*

CLAUSEWITZ'S DISTINCTION BETWEEN projecting power in general and concentrating it at a particular point (see quote above) is fundamental to both military and business strategy. As presented in this chapter, these two approaches to exerting power are also central to the strategic maneuvering of many healthcare organizations. Power strategies are further differentiated by the way power is amassed. Some organizations expand by increasing the number of facilities or locations within the same business, while others grow by combining different kinds of businesses. Whichever pathway is taken, most organizations quickly discover that with growth they must redistribute responsibilities for strategy between business units and corporate headquarters. This is because corporate strategy varies, depending on the size and mix of businesses and markets combined within an organization. Furthermore, it is not always obvious when a shift in corporate strategy is merited. As a result, overlaps between corporate and business unit strategies are common, especially in the early stages of organizational growth, a lesson many healthcare organizations learned in the 1990s.

Because of the diverse ways by which organizations pursue power strategies, this chapter covers the topic in four parts. First, we apply Clausewitz's distinction between overall and concentrated power to healthcare strategy. Second, we conceptualize the types of power strategy that are commonly in use today. Third, we explore the important relationship between corporate strategy and alternative forms of power strategy. Finally, we consider the possibility that organizations follow a fairly predictable pattern of growth as they evolve from employing one type of power strategy to another.

ABSOLUTE POWER VERSUS RELATIVE POWER

Clausewitz's (2000, 427) assertion—"the best strategy is always to be very strong, first of all generally, then at the decisive point"—suggests that power can be applied generally, reflecting the overall or absolute force available to a competitor, or relatively, concentrating force in a particular situation. (See Strategy Note 7.1 for two examples of how relative power was applied in U.S. military history.)

Figure 7.1 graphically illustrates the difference between absolute and relative powers. As shown, *absolute power* draws on the obvious advantages of being categorically large. The overall scale of an organization is an indicator of its level of absolute power. The buildup of conglomerate organizations in the first half of the twentieth century, for example, was motivated by assumptions that larger organizational forms provided significant advantages that were unavailable to smaller rivals. Increases in absolute power are assumed to be associated with gains in economies of scale or scope and market clout. They are also assumed to increase an organization's ability to spread risk, create and project brand identities, derive synergies from diverse businesses, and pursue other advantages that might be correlated with larger organizational scale.

Relative power derives advantages from the concentration of forces within specific markets or points in time. An organization's market share is an appropriate indicator of its relative power, specifying how "big" an organization is relative to its competitors in a given market. Relative power can provide considerable advantages to a competitor, even if it is not large in absolute terms. Small organizations (in absolute terms) can dominate larger ones within individual markets; in fact, this is often the case in the hospital sector. On the other hand, an absolutely large competitor, even if it does not enjoy a high share in a given market, can draw on such advantages as overall mass, deep pockets, and economies of scale to overwhelm a locally dominant rival. The importance of relative power is illustrated by the government's emphasis on antitrust enforcement to

Figure 7.1. Two Ways to Project Market Power

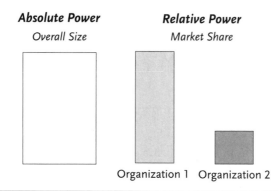

Absolute Power
Overall Size

Relative Power
Market Share

Organization 1   Organization 2

curb excessive concentrations of power within individual markets. Individual competitors that possess high market shares can significantly restrain the overall competitiveness of markets. On the other side of the ledger, competitors are usually well aware that relative power can produce sizable advantages in local competition.

Absolute and Relative Powers in Healthcare

Both approaches to building power—absolute and relative—played prominent roles in the strategies adopted by healthcare providers, insurers, and suppliers in the tumultuous 1990s. In that period, hospitals formed into local strategic alliances and physicians joined ever-larger group practices. Managed care companies even got into the act by selectively merging with direct competitors, thereby not only eliminating rivals but also building up absolute and relative powers, the latter at the local market level.

The value of possessing absolute power is illustrated by Columbia/HCA's dramatic series of acquisitions in the 1990s. During that time, rumors were rampant that Columbia/HCA "had been in town," trying to purchase this or that hospital or physician practice in the area. Fears that Columbia/HCA might become a major local player, for example, stimulated the 1995 merger in Jacksonville, Florida, of two religious-based systems—one owned by the then Daughters of Charity (now called Ascension) and the other by the Baptist Health System. Interestingly, this merger came apart in 2000 after the perceived threat dissipated, leaving the merged companies to struggle with deep and essentially irreconcilable internal conflicts. (Although Columbia/HCA achieved considerable power

STRATEGY NOTE 7.1. RELATIVE POWER AND THE U.S. MILITARY: TWO EXAMPLES

Example 1: Lee's Strategy at Gettysburg
Source: Shaara, M. 1974. *The Killer Angels*. New York: Ballantine Books.

At the battle at Gettysburg, we see a clear distinction between the applications of absolute and relative powers. The Union Army was both larger and better equipped than the Army of the South. Despite this advantage, the South frequently out-maneuvered the North and thereby prolonged the civil war. One important strategy used by the South to gain advantage was to concentrate its forces against weak points in the Union Army. But this did not always work, as Robert E. Lee's experience at Gettysburg demonstrated so plainly. Lee tried twice to concentrate his forces in that battle, but, unfortunately for the South, both attempts failed.

On the first day of battle, Lee attempted to move around the left flank of the Union Army to envelop it and to attack it from the rear. By attacking from the side and rear, he hoped to gain a power advantage that he would not otherwise enjoy were he to attack directly all along the line of battle. The attack that day, known as the battle of Little Big Top, failed at the last moment, when the Union defenders, rushing the Confederates with bayonets drawn, caused the Southern warriors to flee in the face of this surprising maneuver.

On the second day, Lee revised his strategy. Again, he attempted to concentrate his forces at a particular point, this time by attacking with full force the center of the Union line. He had hoped that by doing so, the Confederates would break through the line, divide the Union forces into two, and attack on two flanks at once. First, Lee directed his artillery to bombard the center. Then, after softening up the Union forces (so he mistakenly thought), he commanded his cavalry and foot soldiers to rush the center. Sometimes referred to as Picket's Charge, this strategy produced one of the major losses for the

South in the war. Ironically, this was not a failure of the concept of concentration as a power strategy, but simply a critical mistake in generalship. Lee failed to take into account the obvious danger inherent in charging across an open field, no matter how much power his soldiers poured into the attack. As a result, many Confederate soldiers were killed at Gettysburg, and Lee's troops were forced to retreat back to the South.

Example 2: Eishenhower's Strategy on D-Day

Source: Ambrose, S.E. 1994. *D-Day, June 6, 1944: The Climatic Battle of World War II*. New York: Simon & Schuster.

Dwight D. Eisenhower also decided to concentrate power on that most significant of all World War II battles—D-Day. Having invaded and conquered France, the German Army fully expected that the Allied Forces would soon counterattack. They thus built strong defenses up and down the coast of France. This too was an application of a relative power strategy, the Germans having concluded that the key point of defense was along the coastal line of France. Eisenhower knew full well what the Germans were doing, so he decided to concentrate his forces at an even narrower point along that line: Normandy.

Paralleling Lee's Gettysburg strategy, the D-Day battle began with a massive bombardment of German defenses, followed by an unremitting movement of light infantry, tanks, and other weaponry onto the beaches of Normandy. The scale of the attack was unprecedented in modern military history. Approximately 130,000 soldiers, 12,000 aircraft, and 5,000 ships were involved in this historic confrontation. Both sides lost many lives on that fateful day, but the invasion accomplished its objective: it enabled Allied Forces to penetrate France; splinter the German forces; and drive them, over time, out of France. In this instance, the strategy of concentrating power altered the course of history.

nationally and in Florida, it gained little relative power in Jacksonville.) The formation of other large multihospital systems (e.g., the merger between AMI and NME that formed Tenet), mergers among managed care companies (e.g., between Aetna, U.S. Healthcare, and Prudential HealthCare), and mergers and acquisitions among distributor companies (e.g., between Cardinal and Allegiance) are examples of organizations pursuing absolute power.

Over the last several decades, and especially in the 1990s, not-for-profit hospital systems tended to favor relative power; as a result, many have emerged as leading players within their individual markets. A number of not for profits also moved beyond their local boundaries, although, in contrast to the for profits, they tended to move into markets that are geographically nearby (such strategies are explored further in Chapter 8). Many provider systems began flexing their significant gains in relative power by negotiating aggressively with managed care companies. For example, the Center for Studying Health System Change (HSC) (Strunk, Devers, and Hurley 2001) found that an increasing number of contract disputes erupted between health plans and providers (hospitals and physicians) at the local market level. HSC observed that some providers, relying on strong market positions (relative power), threatened to terminate their participation in the health plans if their payment demands were not met. Many hospital systems were thus using their local strength to counter the greater absolute power of the managed care companies.

Absolute and relative powers can be pursued independently or simultaneously. From the 1970s through the 1980s, for-profit organizations tended to rely exclusively on absolute power, seeking acquisitions and building small hospitals in selected high-growth areas. For these organizations, local dominance was of far less strategic importance than capturing prize locations across the country. Exceptions existed, of course. In the 1980s, the Humana Hospital Corporation placed a high level of emphasis on achieving dominant positions in local markets while continuing to build its overall corporate mass. In the 1990s, most for-profit organizations, following the lead of not for profits, began emphasizing relative power as well, a major strategy pursued by Columbia/HCA in concert with its pursuit of absolute power strategy nationwide.

TYPES OF POWER STRATEGIES

The four major types of power strategy differ chiefly by whether the expansion combines similar or different businesses. This is an important distinction because the former draws heavily on the advantages of scale and learning and the latter on the advantages of scale and scope. The four types are as follows:

Same Businesses
1. *Horizontal expansion*: expansion in the scale of existing business activities (e.g., the merger of two or more hospitals)

Different Businesses (also referred to as diversification)
1. *Vertical integration*: the combination and coordination of businesses that share input-output relationships (e.g., integrating hospital and managed care companies)
2. *Horizontal integration*: the combination and coordination of different types of businesses that are not vertically related (e.g., jointly managing hotel and hospital companies)
3. *Portfolio*: the combination and financial coordination of different types of businesses; the exclusive focus on financial is the primary difference between portfolio and horizontal integration

The term "horizontal" describes two different power strategies. The first, horizontal expansion, applies to growth within the same business area; the second, horizontal integration, applies to the combination and integration of different businesses.

Global diversification can be added to these four types, a type that has become so important in many industries over the past several decades (Bourgeois, Duhaime, and Stimpert 1999). A few healthcare organizations provide services beyond the borders of the United States: HCA currently owns hospitals in England and Switzerland, Tenet owns a hospital in Spain, and many major manufacturers of healthcare products are active internationally. Global diversification is not included in our list of power strategies, however, simply because it is such an unlikely strategic option for the vast majority of provider organizations.

Horizontal expansion is indisputably the most common power strategy pursued by competitors across industries, and healthcare providers are no different in this regard. Horizontal expansion occurs when organizations seek advantage by expanding within the same business area (e.g., within acute care), either by penetrating existing markets or expanding into new markets. The reasons that horizontal expansion is so important are simple. First, growth in nearly any form provides gains in both organizational scale and market power. Second, growth within an organization's existing business areas is generally the least risky of the four strategies. Organizations know their own businesses, the structures of their markets, and the capabilities of the players (i.e., buyers, sellers, competitors); thus, they are likely to pursue horizontal expansion as a first line of offense (or defense). This assumes, of course, that the market structures in which these organizations operate support horizontal expansion. Some fragmented markets, for example, might not support the buildup of power as a workable approach to achieving competitive advantage (see Chapter 4).

Vertical integration achieves growth by combining buyers and sellers into the same organization. A seller acquiring or entering into the industry of a buyer engages in forward integration (the reverse is backward integration). Even though this strategy combines different businesses, organizations seeking to integrate vertically presumably have considerable knowledge about their target acquisitions. As buyers from or sellers to targeted acquisitions, they are usually in a position to observe and experience first hand the target's business practices. Vertical integration increases organizational mass, opens up opportunities for organizations to manage more efficiently and effectively their buyer/seller transactions, and enables organizations to predict more accurately downstream (forward integration) or upstream (backward integration) market behaviors and conditions. (Vertical integration is discussed in detail in Chapter 9.)

Horizontal integration combines different businesses, whether they are similar (or related) or dissimilar (or unrelated) to one another. Such businesses are combined for two primary reasons. First, as with the other power strategies, horizontal integration increases organizational mass, thereby increasing gains in organizational scale and power. Second, by definition, horizontal integration opens up opportunities for interorganizational synergies. Vertical integration can be seen as a subset of horizontal integration because both strategies seek advantages from the combination of different business entities. Vertical integration is separately identified, however, simply because it is such a significant and distinctive form of multibusiness combination. Because vertical integration joins buyers and sellers, it facilitates better management of product flows, market exchanges and negotiations, and distribution channels, advantages that are not generally available with horizontal integration.

Portfolio also combines different businesses, but it has far less expectation for interorganizational integration. Portfolio focuses distinctly and specifically on financial coordination. It provides the advantages of greater organizational scale and opportunities to reallocate resources across owned businesses and to improve subsidiary performance through corporate financial monitoring and control. Portfolio also offers the advantages of spreading risk across different businesses, each of which faces distinctive strategic, environmental, and financial conditions. Apart from presenting opportunities for increased mass and financial synergies, portfolio provides little rationale for organizations to engage in this form of strategy.

The use of horizontal integration and portfolio (which are commonly referred to as diversification strategies) is nearly nonexistent among health-care providers, although examples exist within the healthcare supply sector. However, as healthcare provider organizations continue to grow in size and complexity and as their corporate capabilities mature, they will begin to pursue horizontal integration or portfolio strategies.

Identifying the Power Strategy Applied

Despite the seemingly clear distinctions between the four power strategies, determining which strategy is being applied in actual practice is not easy. One version of a multibusiness strategy can be categorized as vertical integration, horizontal integration, or portfolio (or any combination of the three), depending on the particulars, if the strategy is consummated. An example of this is the attempt in 1984 by HCA and the American Hospital Supply Corporation (AHSC) to merge. To judge which power strategy was involved in this proposed merger requires having more information about the underlying rationale for the merger.

The proposed merger attempted to integrate AHSC, the leading supplier of medical/surgical products to hospitals at that time, and HCA, the largest for-profit, multihospital system in the country. Upon its announcement, warning bells went off on both Wall Street and main street, the intensity of which ultimately prevented the merger from being consummated. This merger was seen as a bad idea for many reasons, not the least of which was an expected negative reaction by many HCA competitors (who perceived this as a vertical strategy). Analysts feared that those competitors would respond by switching supply contracts from AHSC to one of its rivals. In fact, the number two distributor at the time, Owens & Minor, considered the announcement of the merger to be very good news. As HCA rivals turned away from AHSC, Owens & Minor fully expected to see a major increase in its contracts with hospitals (especially not-for-profit hospitals and systems). Facing criticism from all sides, HCA and AHSC called off the merger. A year later, AHSC merged instead with Baxter Travenol, a major manufacturer of hospital supplies; this merger resulted in a mixed vertical and horizontal integration form of business combination. Ironically, this merger was later undone when, more than a decade later, Baxter spun off a major part of its distribution business and formed Allegiance (which has since merged [under horizontal integration strategy] with Cardinal, a major pharmaceutical distribution company).

So what was the strategic rationale for the proposed HCA-AHSC merger? It could not have been horizontal expansion because the proposed merger involved two very different businesses. At first blush, it seems to have been vertical integration, as HCA was a major buyer of supplies distributed by AHSC. However, it can qualify as vertical only if the primary rationale for the combination were to reduce the transaction costs associated with buying and selling between the two organizations. The merger could have been horizontal integration as well, if coordinated channel management were not the prime consideration but other forms of integration were (e.g., combining information system infrastructures, merging marketing and business development activities). It could have been a portfolio strategy if the primary rationale were not integration at all but to improve the use and distribution of funds across the two organizations. Anecdotal evidence suggests that all three reasons played a part in the initial thinking. With respect to portfolio, for example, AHSC was an organization that enjoyed a dominating position in distribution but had limited prospects for further growth. HCA, on the other hand, was perceived at the time to have a limitless growth trajectory. By the mid-1980s, HCA owned or managed approximately 450 hospitals and its prospects for further growth were bright. Further growth for HCA depended, to a considerable extent, on gaining access to additional funding sources; AHSC could have been that source. In other words, AHSC was a possible cash cow that could have helped to fund HCA's expansion through intracorporate transfers.

CORPORATE STRATEGY VERSUS BUSINESS UNIT STRATEGY

Before we delve further into power strategies, a distinction has to be drawn between corporate and business unit strategies. *Corporate strategy* deals with the whole of organizations, including the multiple businesses and interrelationships that exist or might exist among them (as determined by careful management assessments). *Business unit strategy*, on the other hand, is restricted to the strategic agenda of single businesses. It therefore focuses directly on how a given business might gain competitive advantage over its rivals. Corporate strategy is broader and more comprehensive, while business unit strategy is more focused on the specifics of the competitive battlefield. Because corporate strategy extracts advantage from the combination of businesses owned by an organization, power strategies (each of which involves combinations of businesses) fall mostly within the domain of corporate strategy.

Corporate and business unit strategies can overlap to a considerable degree, a problem that has been particularly acute for many not-for-profit hospital systems. The merger of, say, three hospitals in a local market might necessitate the formation of a corporate structure to coordinate the hospitals and their strategies; in this case, each hospital is treated as a separate business unit. On the other hand, because the combined hospitals share a high strategic interest in local competition, the three might instead be configured into a single business unit. In fact, for this very purpose, a number of hospitals have merged, even after becoming members of the same organization. In any case, even if a corporate structure were formed in this instance, corporate likely would not be able to avoid becoming actively involved in setting and coordinating local market strategies for each of the combined hospitals because of the close geographic proximities and high shared strategic interests.

Also, a multibusiness organization likely might not need to form a corporate layer. Such has been the case for many hospitals, as they have steadily moved considerably beyond the provision of strictly acute care services. Many hospitals across the country now provide rehabilitation, psychiatric, long-term, ambulatory, emergency, and various other kinds and levels of care in addition to acute care. Despite such growth in product/business diversity, many of these hospitals have adjusted and added to their existing management capacities rather than establish independent corporate entities. In most such situations, the core hospital agenda has dominated the strategic thinking. On the other hand, some hospitals have evolved to the point that they need independent corporate and business unit layers. Unfortunately, no clear formula exists that reliably signals the stage in organizational growth at which an independent corporate structure is required, regardless of whether an organization is involved in multimarket or multibusiness expansion activities.

The Domain of Corporate Strategy

Traditionally, corporate strategy has been relegated to financing and choosing businesses—that is, to deciding whether to keep existing businesses, whether to enter new businesses, and how to allocate funds among the organization's businesses (see Colley, Doyle, and Hardie 2002). As such, corporate strategy has had little to do with directing, integrating, or deciding competitive strategies for the subsidiaries. This restrictive conceptualization springs directly from the roots of corporate strategy—that is, from the strategic rationale provided for the conglomerate (portfolio) business model. Because conglomerates run collections of diverse businesses, their corporations generally delegate responsibility for establishing and running business unit strategies to their individual units. The role of the corporate in such cases is typically limited to choosing, financing, and monitoring functions.

The analytic tools designed to assist in corporate strategic decision making reflect this concept of the corporate role. The classic portfolio-analysis grid conceived by Boston Consulting Group (BCG), for example, served precisely this limited purpose (see Strategic Tool C at the end of this chapter for a discussion of the BCG Grid and other portfolio analysis tools). The *BCG Grid* was designed specifically to assist in the financial analysis of an organization's businesses. Organizations using a portfolio model, by definition, are not involved in extracting synergies or facilitating integration across owned business units.

Moving Beyond Portfolio

More recently, some strategy experts have called for greater emphasis on integrating businesses across an organization's portfolio. Porter (1985), for example, has suggested that organizations should take care in selecting businesses so that added advantage can be extracted out of the joint administration. He argued that financial management of a portfolio of businesses amounted to little more than managing a stock portfolio and that the only difference between these two is that the corporation owned its particular portfolio of businesses. Wouldn't it be better, he asked, to involve the corporation more directly in the strategic realm of its owned businesses? Porter based his criticism on empirical findings in which conglomerate organizations appeared, on average, to contribute little to the strategic performance of their subsidiaries. In his own research, he evaluated 33 large conglomerates from 1950 to 1986; he came up with the following conclusion (Porter 1998, 120–21):

I found that on average corporations divested more than half their acquisitions in new industries and more than 60 percent of their acquisitions in entirely new fields. Fourteen companies left more than 70 percent of all the acquisitions they had made in new fields. The track record in unrelated acquisitions is even worse—the average divestment rate is a startling 74 percent.... My data give a stark indication of the failure of corporate strategies. Of the thirty-three companies, six had been taken over as my study was being completed. Only the lawyers, investment bankers, and original sellers have prospered in most of these acquisitions, not the shareholders.

A better approach, Porter suggested, is for corporations to become more deeply involved in assisting their subsidiaries in their attempts to achieve competitive advantage. To do this, corporations needed to capture the advantages of scale and scope that presumably are available if related businesses were integrated, advantages that, in effect, come from horizontal expansion, vertical integration, or horizontal integration.

Porter (1998, 131–45) then identified four alternative roles that corporations might take as they engage in multibusiness activities:

1. *Portfolio management*: The traditional role whereby corporations merely regulate the finances of their owned subsidiaries.
2. *Restructuring*: In the earliest phases of business acquisition, corporate moves beyond financial management to restructure the acquired business (e.g., by changing the management team, modifying its strategy, building improved information systems). This involvement is generally seen as a one-time event, with the corporation returning to its relatively passive role of financial management once the restructuring is completed.
3. *Transferring information*: This role assumes that the corporation is able to transfer valuable information (e.g., about distribution channels, use of technology, management tricks and tools) among business units. For sharing opportunities to exist, the businesses not only need to be sufficiently related but the information to be shared also has to be both of strategic value and proprietary. Furthermore, a more involved corporate role is justified only if valued sharing can be extended well beyond a one-time event.
4. *Sharing activities*: Under this role, the corporation facilitates the sharing and integration of important "activities" performed by the

owned businesses; this role involves more than the transfer of knowledge or one-time transfers of knowledge or skills. For an interorganizational coordination to be successful, sharing must produce economies of scale. Otherwise, the value of combining/sharing activities might not outweigh the costs of coordination. Also, the shared activities have to be important strategically—that is, they have to make a difference in generating competitive advantage and have to be inimitable to competition.

Multibusiness Integration in Healthcare

The efforts of many hospitals to form integrated systems are generally consistent with Porter's fourth role (sharing activities). At the beginning of the 1990s, many organizations held to the view that if they combined physician practices, hospitals, nursing homes, home health businesses, and other healthcare businesses, they would achieve significant gains in efficiencies, quality, access to care, and competitive advantage. They assumed that physicians especially could benefit from the sophisticated management support systems available within hospitals. They expected that patient flows and patient information could be managed more efficiently through the integration of diverse provider types. Also, they assumed that by combining locally, hospitals could share the expensive and often underutilized high-tech resources needed to provide tertiary and quaternary care. The fact that many hospitals experienced significant difficulties in extracting real and continuing advantages from integration speaks volumes about the challenges inherent in multibusiness combinations.

Also in the 1990s, several of the major players in the supply distribution sector assumed that significant advantages could be obtained by pursuing integrative strategies. The key idea was that because the providers were becoming integrated at the local level, the distribution companies should pursue a parallel course to better serve the needs of the new, more complex systems. Specifically, as illustrated in Figure 7.2, they considered three forms of integration:

1. Integration across market segments
2. Integration across product categories
3. Integration using information technology and other technologies

McKesson Corporation, based in San Francisco, took the lead by moving in all three of these directions. By the end of the 1970s, McKesson had

Figure 7.2. Integrative Strategies in the Supply Distribution Sector

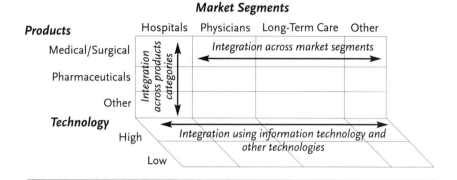

become a leading distributor of drugs, alcoholic beverages, and chemicals in the United States. It also emerged as a major distributor of milk-based products and processed water. As it moved into the 1980s, however, McKesson divested many of its businesses and focused directly on health-care supply distribution. In the 1990s, its multibusiness focus returned. First, McKesson, primarily a pharmaceutical distribution company (a single product area), acquired General Medical (GM), a distributor of medical/surgical products. At that time, GM was distributing medical/surgical products to three market segments: (1) hospitals (GM was the third largest distributor to this segment), (2) physicians (GM was the leading distributor for this segment), and (3) long-term care (GM was a leading distributor here). By combining pharmaceutical and medical/surgical distribution, McKesson hoped to sell an "integrated" capability (integrated across products and segments) to the integrated delivery systems being formed. Thus, it positioned itself to provide a full line of healthcare products, from drugs to diapers, to all of the segments represented in the forming integrated delivery systems.

Second, McKesson made a critical assumption that distribution was increasingly becoming an information-processing business. Therefore, it acquired a leading healthcare software and consulting company by the name of HBOC. Again, McKesson's underlying rationale was integration. It assumed that the distribution and information business units could share information, distribution channels, and product design strategies in developing an outsourcing and supply management product that could be marketed to providers. The jury is still out on whether McKesson's integration strategies will in the long run provide a sustainable advantage.

In any case, the McKesson approach is fully consistent with Porter's fourth level of corporate involvement in maximizing competitive advantage through interorganizational coordination.

The foregoing examples demonstrate how corporate strategy in healthcare is viewed as more than merely choosing and financing multiple provider units. Most healthcare organizations, of course, needed no convincing of this fact. The field is heavily invested in finding ways to rationalize (through system integration) the otherwise fragmented "system" of delivery.

Defining Corporate Strategy

To define corporate strategy, we need to take this broad view: corporate strategy extends well beyond choosing from among and managing the finances of individual business units. This view recognizes that existing interdependencies among business units, if properly arranged and managed by an effective corporate leadership, can be translated into measurable gains in competitive advantage, for both the individual and the collective units. In many respects, corporate strategy and business unit strategy are similar: both seek to build competitive advantage. The primary difference between them is that corporate strategy seeks competitive advantage by working on the interrelationships between units, and business strategy focuses directly on market rivalry at the business unit level. Given that, here is a definition of corporate strategy:

> Corporate strategies are those key concepts and ideas that relate to the selection, financing, and integration of business units for the purpose of gaining and sustaining competitive advantage for the organization as a whole.

This definition directly parallels the definition of strategy developed in Chapter 1. Its focus is conceptual, and the focus is on gaining and sustaining competitive advantage. The key difference between corporate and business unit strategies, however, remains.

Figure 7.3 presents the arenas of corporate and business units as they relate to power strategies. As shown, business unit strategies fall within the single business category, within the realm of horizontal expansion. The shaded areas in horizontal expansion, however, suggest that as one moves from single to multimarkets (or from single to multiple facilities), the need for a separate corporate structure arises. The white boxes represent the arenas of vertical and horizontal integration. This is where different businesses

Figure 7.3. Arenas of Corporate and Business Unit Strategies

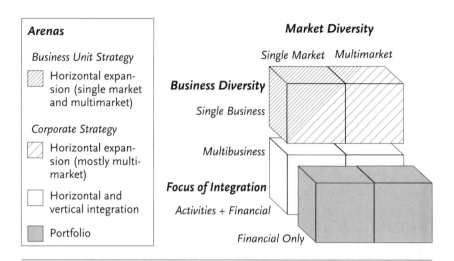

are managed, with emphasis on both financial and other kinds of synergies. Finally, the gray boxes represent portfolio strategy, which is distinguished from vertical and horizontal integrations by its exclusive focus on financial integration.

Given that both strategies are focused on gaining competitive advantage, conflicts between them will inevitably arise. The greater the emphasis on interdependencies, the greater those overlaps will be.

Sources of Advantage at Corporate and Business Unit Levels

To what extent each of the five sources of competitive advantage applies to corporate and business unit strategies must be considered at this point. Undoubtedly, all sources apply to individual business units. But do they apply as well to corporate strategy? The answer is yes; however, as suggested in Table 7.1, the relative importance of each source might vary between business unit and corporate levels. Perhaps the greatest difference is the degree to which positioning serves as an important source of advantage at the business unit level. Positioning is obviously significant at the business unit level because direct rivalry at this level often involves jockeying for desirable cost, quality, service, location, and other positions. By contrast, corporations tend to be somewhat less visible to individual consumers or competitors and thus are less likely to turn to positioning as a source of advantage. Consumers might be aware, for example, that PepsiCo owns

Table 7.1. Relative Importance of Sources of Advantage, by Organization Level

		Level	
			Strategic
		Corporate	Business Unit
Source	Power	High	High
	Pace	Medium	High
	Position	Low	Medium
	Potential	High	High
	Performance	High	High

Pepsi, but they are less likely to know that PepsiCo also owns Frito-Lay, Gatorade, Tropicana, and Quaker Foods. Positioning is undoubtedly not a key source of competitive advantage for PepsiCo corporate, although it certainly is for its subsidiaries and their respective product lines.

Positioning may not be especially useful for Hillenbrand Industries either. Hillenbrand, a publically traded holding company headquartered in Batesville, Indiana, owns Hill-Rom (also based in Batesville), the leading producer and distributor of advanced healthcare beds, therapy surfaces, headwall systems, and other patient and operating room equipment. Significantly, Hill-Rom's bed systems enjoy an overwhelmingly dominant market share within the acute care hospital sector. Positioning also played a key role in Hill-Rom's rise to dominance in its markets. Hill-Rom places a very high value on knowing and responding to its customers and their changing needs. Hill-Rom and its bed and care systems are widely recognized by providers, especially within the acute care sector, but Hillenbrand, the parent company, is not. The identity of the parent also does not contribute to the positioning of its other two businesses—Batesville Casket Company and Forethought Financial Services, Inc. Hillenbrand is a holding company and as such serves primarily to manage the overall finances of its subsidiaries. Beyond that, it is little involved in the day-to-day competitive struggles of its subsidiaries. In sum, positioning is simply not an important source of competitive advantage for Hillenbrand; for that matter, neither is integration across the business units, which is consistent with it being a conglomerate or portfolio model firm.

In contrast to Hillenbrand, many examples exist of companies that have well-established positions at the corporate level. Consider, for example, how important the names General Electric, General Motors, Microsoft, IBM, and Johnson & Johnson are to their various product lines and businesses.

In terms of healthcare providers, companies such as Intermountain Health Care, Sutter Health, Sentara, and Kaiser Permanente all have well-established corporate positions that serve powerfully to reinforce the positions of their respective business units. In many such cases, the position of the corporate, not the business unit, is what makes the competitive difference. Also, the positions of many provider systems are grounded in the reputations for quality and technological sophistication of their hub hospitals, and such is the case with The Cleveland Clinic, Mayo Clinic, Johns Hopkins Hospital & Health System, and Shands HealthCare. Despite these examples, most provider organizations do not emphasize their corporate identities, which is the case for most large for-profit organizations. Today, HCA, given the negative publicity its corporate entity received in the 1990s, explicitly downplays its corporate identity or corporate positioning.

The remaining four sources of advantage—power, potential, performance, and pace—are clearly important at both the corporate and business unit levels. Power is the sine qua non of competitive advantage at the corporate level, and it is highly critical at the business unit level as well. Acquiring and integrating internal resources, processes, and capabilities (potential and performance) are also critically important at both levels. Furthermore, corporate entities play crucial roles in promoting performance objectives within their subsidiary businesses. Also, they often address the timing and aggressiveness (pace) of strategic action as they make acquisitions, divest businesses, and set funding priorities for and approve the overall strategies of their subsidiaries.

Efforts to integrate at the local level, especially, force many strategic issues up the organizational hierarchy. This can create some confusion about the respective roles of corporate and business units in the area of strategy, but that responsibility for integration undoubtedly falls primarily within the corporate domain, which includes locally organized hospital-based systems.

SEQUENCE OF STRATEGIC GROWTH

Finally, we consider whether organizations follow sequences or typical pathways of strategic growth in their pursuit of power strategy options, or whether their choices of strategic options are essentially idiosyncratic. Some important research has been done on the stages of growth through which organizations pass. Much of the emphasis has been on the relationship between organizational structure and strategy. Alfred Chandler's (1962) longitudinal studies of large organizations as they evolved through the first half of the twentieth century laid the groundwork for this kind of analysis. He found that as organizations changed strategies, they implemented new organizational structures. Chandler also identified three stages of organizational evolution. The first was an entrepreneurial stage, in which the leader-entrepreneur made all of the key decisions and in which strategy focused on single product areas. The second stage focused on both market and product development. Here, the organization tended to emphasize functional divisions within the organization (see Chapter 10), with a focus on capturing the advantages of integration. In the third stage, organizations had diversified into related or unrelated businesses. At this point, decentralized, multidivisional organizational structures were needed given the limited role corporations played in both the management and strategy formation.

A number of scholars built on the groundbreaking work of Chandler (Buchele 1967; Collins and Moore 1970; Salter 1970; Scott and Bruce 1987; Thain 1969). Milton Leontiades (1980) provided one of the more logical conceptualizations of the stages of growth. As have others, he suggested that organizations sequence through a series of stages as they grow and mature and consequently as they build the internal capacity needed for strategic change. Specifically, he identified four key stages through which organizations tend to evolve (see Figure 7.4).

As illustrated in the figure, organizations begin by focusing on a single business area, Leontiades's single-business stage (first). With growth, they move on to building product line diversity, the dominant single-business stage (second). Both of these stages involve growth primarily in size. The dominant stage involves some product diversity, but its essential strategic idea is to expand within the initial business area. The first and second stages are consistent with the horizontal expansion strategy.

In the next two stages, organizations move into the multiple businesses arena; here, no one business necessarily dominates an organization. The third and fourth stages reflect the degree to which organizations pursue integration as a strategy or manage their businesses as independent entities. Leontiades is suggesting that organizations are more likely to engage in horizontal expansion first and then, at some point, move to vertical or horizontal integration. Lastly, if at all, organizations might move into portfolio, which is similar to the logic provided by Chandler.

Leontiades reasoned (as indicated in the figure) that the most significant change in stage occurs when organizations shift from horizontal expansion (size growth) to multibusiness strategies (diversity growth).

Figure 7.4. Leontiades's Stages of Growth

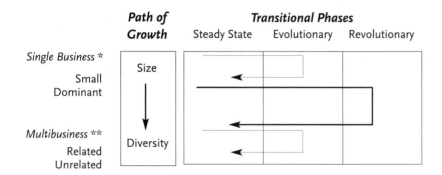

Path of Growth   *Transitional Phases* — Steady State, Evolutionary, Revolutionary

Single Business *
    Small
    Dominant

Multibusiness **
    Related
    Unrelated

Size → Diversity

* The arena of horizontal expansion strategy
** The arena of vertical integration, horizontal integration, and portfolio
Revolutionary ─────────────▶

Source: Adapted with permission from Leontiades, M. 1980. *Strategies for Diversification and Change*, 98. Boston: Little Brown and Co. Copyright by Milton Leontiades.

Movement into diverse businesses shifts organizations higher up on the learning curve and as a result increases their overall risk, at least initially. Because of this, he suggested, significant, possibly revolutionary changes in management, organizational structure, culture, and board composition might be needed as organizations move from size to diversity expansion.

Within each of the two general approaches to growth, the risks involved in shifting between the stages would be far less. Accordingly, Leontiades suggested that shifts in structures, leadership, and so on, would be less dramatic (more evolutionary), although significant changes in these areas might still be needed. Executives familiar with smaller, single-business management, for example, might not have the requisite skills to coordinate complex business arrangements or to modify the organizational structure to ensure that the added business lines are administered properly. In such situations, changes in leadership (and possibly in board composition and structure) might be needed.

Many hospital organizations moved from single to dominant business forms in the 1990s, and some even moved into the true multibusiness arena (e.g., vertical integration). However, that all of them made the needed adjustments in management and structure prescribed by

Leontiades is not obvious. When the Minneapolis-based HealthSpan (a hospital company) merged with Medica (a managed care company) forming Allina (discussed in Chapter 6), for example, a compromised, rather than a radically new structure, appeared to have been adopted. In working out the details of the merger, it was agreed that the prior executives of the two organizations would stay on in a kind of shared leadership arrangement. In other words, they did not recruit a new management team to run this very different and much more complex (vertically integrated) organizational form. Obviously, this was a halfway solution, a resolution between the discordant institutionalized powers within the merging companies. Failure to commit to a major restructuring of the management team and the organizational structure might have contributed to the demise of Allina. The merger lasted eight years, coming undone in 2001.

Making the needed adjustments in structure is likely to be a problem many provider systems will encounter whenever they shift through the stages of growth. Much of the difficulty here can be attributed to the historically grounded and often very powerful institutional sources of resistance. A merger between two religious-affiliated organizations, for example, might face some considerable hurdles when the two entities attempt to formulate appropriate administrative structures. The combination of physician and hospital organizations can run directly into well-recognized struggles over control. Movement through the Leontiades stages of growth can be more challenging for the provider sector than expected.

Stages of Growth in Healthcare

Combining the Leontiades stages with Ansoff's (1965) well-known growth matrix illustrates some of the distinctive patterns of growth that are followed by provider organizations. As shown in Table 7.2, Ansoff suggested that growth strategies can be differentiated by whether they involve movement into new markets or new products. This leads to four major growth options:

1. Market penetration
2. Market expansion (the equivalent of horizontal expansion)
3. Product development
4. Diversification (vertical integration, horizontal integration, and portfolio)

Table 7.2. Evolution of Hospital Strategies: Integrating Leontiades's Stages of Growth Model and Ansoff's Growth Matrix

Traditional Business Model

Products

Markets		Old	New
	Old	Market Penetration	Product Development
	New	Market Expansion	Diversification

Naïve Hospital Model

Products

Markets		Old	New
	Old	Market Penetration	Product Development
	New	Market Expansion	Diversification

Community Hospital Model

Products

Markets		Old	New
	Old	Market Penetration	Product Development
	New	Market Expansion	Diversification

Not-for-Profit Hospital Model

Products

Markets		Old	New
	Old	Market Penetration	Product Development
	New	Market Expansion	Diversification

Source: Adapted from New Corporate Strategy: An Analytic Approach to Business Policy for Growth and Expansion, by H. I. Ansoff, 109. Copyright © 1965. This material is used by permission of John Wiley & Sons, Inc.

The first three are consistent with Leontiades's single-business-unit (small and dominant) stages, and the last is consistent with his multi-business (related and unrelated) stages.

Using this framework, we can illustrate the stages logic developed earlier. Organizations begin with market penetration and move down the learning curve of their existing businesses. A hospital, for example, can do this by expanding the capacity of its facility or combining with another hospital within its local market. At some point, organizations can be expected to take advantage of gains in learning and scale by moving those same businesses into new markets. In time and with growth in size, management capacity, and resources, organizations might begin moving into Leontiades's second stage, which is continue growing the existing business but also gradually add product lines and maybe smaller related businesses. Further growth after that might take organizations in a major new direction—into multibusiness activities, which includes the last two stages identified by Leontiades.

This pathway of growth is illustrated in the first diagram in Table 7.2, labeled the "traditional business model." This model appears to have been followed by for-profit hospital organizations over the years and by the physician practice management companies in the 1990s. These organizations moved directly into new market expansion (size expansion in space) before engaging in many product developments and, certainly, before considering diversity expansion. The Catholic systems have also actively pursued multimarket expansion, which to a large extent reflects religious objectives.

Most not-for-profit systems, by contrast, tend to follow a distinctly different pathway to growth. Virtually all not-for-profit hospitals have engaged actively and locally in product development; with a few exceptions, most have been reluctant to expand beyond the borders of their local markets, preferring instead to combine with other hospitals and to engage in product development, which are all local. This approach is the "community hospital model" in the figure. In the late 1970s, as the environment grew increasingly hostile, many not-for-profit hospitals and systems even entertained diversification as a strategic option, still resisting market expansion; at that time, the fad was to attend seminars on diversification. This tendency is illustrated in the figure as the "naïve hospital model."

As the 1990s hit, not-for-profit hospitals became more involved in multihospital and multimarket combinations. This general movement outside of local markets is represented in the figure as the "not-for-profit hospital model." In this and other chapters, we offer some reasons that not-for-profit systems might not have given as much priority to multimarket expansion as would be consistent with the traditional business model. They appear to have stayed at home, so to speak, because of their community orientations and missions, the lack of capital required for multimarket expansion, institutional constraints (resistance), or the lack of vision about opportunities for system development.

CONCLUSION

Power strategies are explored in this chapter. Once organizations get involved in multibusiness and multimarket strategies, they discover the need to form corporate structures, which then coordinate and control the owned business units. Sorting out the functions of corporate and business units is especially challenging for healthcare organizations because of very high interorganizational interdependencies. This might be especially true in the field of strategy, which is so intertwined with the pursuit of multiorganizational combinations. Healthcare organizations, like organizations in other industries, appear to be evolving through various stages of business growth, which is a fairly new phenomenon for many organizations, especially not-for-profit hospital providers. Not surprisingly, organizations appear to be moving down somewhat atypical pathways of growth. Most notably, the not for profits tend to avoid multimarket expansion, at least to the degree that other ownership types have pursued this form of growth.

The local orientations of not for profits will, of course, change in time, as they increasingly shift toward more traditional business model patterns of growth (involving expansion into multiple markets). The not-for-profit hospital sector has undergone considerable consolidation in recent years, and many hospitals have formed into multihospital systems, a number of which have expanded into multiple markets, although mostly into areas that are geographically proximate. As not-for-profit systems grow in size and numbers of systems, they can be expected to increasingly develop strategic interests that are independent of their founding hospitals and their leadership. To the extent that this occurs, they will begin to behave more like other businesses, engaging in multimarket and even multibusiness expansion activities. In time, this can further increase the level of consolidation nationally.

REFERENCES

Ambrose, S. E. 1994. *D-Day, June 6, 1944: The Climatic Battle of World War II*. New York: Simon & Schuster.

Ansoff, H. I. 1965. *New Corporate Strategy*. New York: McGraw-Hill.

Bourgeois, L., I. Duhaime, and J. Stimpert. 1999. *Strategic Management: Concepts for Managers*, 2nd ed. Fort Worth, TX: Dryden Press.

Buchele, R. B. 1967. *Business Policy in Growing Firms*. Scranton, PA: Chandler Publishing Company.

Chandler, A. D. 1962. *Strategy and Structure: Chapters in the History of the Industrial Enterprise*. Cambridge, MA: MIT Press.

Clausewitz, K. V. 2000. "Assembly of Forces in Space." In *The Book of War*, edited by C. Carr, 427. New York: Modern Library.

Colley, J. L., J. L. Doyle, and R. D. Hardie. 2002. *Corporate Strategy*. New York: McGraw-Hill.

Collins, O., and D. C. Moore. 1970. *The Organization Makers.* New York: Appleton-Century-Crofts.

Hoffer Schendel, C., and D. Schendel. 1978. *Strategy Formulation: Analytical Concepts.* St. Paul, MN: West Publishing.

Leontiades, M. 1980. *Strategies for Diversification and Change.* Boston: Little Brown and Co.

Porter, M. E. 1985. *Competitive Advantage: Creating and Sustaining Superior Performance.* New York: The Free Press.

————. 1998. *On Competition.* Boston: Harvard Business School Press.

Salter, M. S. 1970. "Stages of Corporate Development." *Journal of Business Policy* 1 (1): 23–27.

Scott, M., and R. Bruce. 1987. "Five Stages of Growth in Small Business." *Long Range Planning* 20 (3): 45–52.

Shaara, M. 1974. *The Killer Angels.* New York: Ballantine Books.

Strunk, B. C., K. Devers, and R. E. Hurley. 2001. "Health Plan-Provider Showdowns on the Rise." [Online article on Center for Studying Health Systems Change web site; retrieved 01/03.] http://www.hschange.com/CONTENT/326/?topic=topic03.

Thain, D. H. 1969. "Stage of Corporate Development." *Business Quarterly* (Winter): 33–45.

STRATEGY TOOL C. PORTFOLIO ANALYSIS TOOLS

One of the major tasks performed at the corporate level of multibusiness or multimarket organizations is to allocate capital among the strategic business units (SBUs). A number of useful tools have been developed for doing this task, most of which use essentially the same logic for assessing SBUs. They evaluate two factors: (1) the broader market environment in which the SBUs are located (market attractiveness) and (2) the competitive position of each SBU. The term "industry attractiveness" is more commonly used outside of healthcare because these tools are typically used to analyze businesses in different industries. However, "market attractiveness" is used for our purposes because the applications in healthcare are usually more micro. We are interested in assessing different businesses or units located in different markets within the same industry.

Historically, such tools were developed for use by portfolio or conglomerate organizations. The primary task of corporate was thus to decide in which businesses to invest (or spin off) and, once those were selected, to allocate resources among them. Although more integrated

Figure 7A. BCG Grid

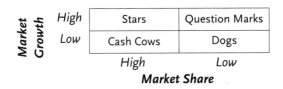

organizations (using horizontal expansion, horizontal integration, or vertical integration) assess more than financial interrelationships, they find these tools to be valuable as well. Three variations on the portfolio analysis tool are discussed here: the BCG Grid, the GE Business Screen, and the mission-based matrix.

The BCG Grid

The most widely recognized, and the least complicated, tool is the Boston Consulting Group (BCG) Grid, which uses two basic variables to analyze SBUs—market share (to analyze SBU strategic positions) and market growth (to analyze the attractiveness of their industries or, in our case, markets). *The BCG Grid* assumes that economies of scale, market power, and other advantages are directly associated with the relative market share enjoyed by an individual business. Also, it assumes that prospects for revenue growth within its markets reflect the most essential feature to be considered when evaluating those markets. The next two tools expand the number of factors to be considered when evaluating markets and SBUs.

An essential element common to all of these tools is that they were designed to assess both the individual SBUs and the collective or portfolio of SBUs. A strategy (or financial) analyst might then use the tool to do the following:

1. *Evaluate the financial viability of each SBU.*
2. *Make strategic choices among the SBUs.*
   - Select SBUs to retain within the portfolio and to sell off ("dogs"—see definitions below)
   - Identify possible acquisition targets
   - Identify SBUs from which funds can be taken ("cash cows") and redistributed to support SBUs that have better long-run prospects for growth and financial return ("stars" and, possibly, "question marks")

3. *Seek a balance among the SBUs, based on the following two dimensions:*
   - Fund-flow balance: SBUs that need (and merit) additional finan-
     cial support ("stars" and, possibly, "question marks") are balanced
     against those that have the capacity to produce excess funds
     ("cash cows").
   - Risk balance: A well-balanced portfolio is one that has a mix of
     high-, medium-, and low-risk SBUs, such that risk can be spread
     across all SBUs.

As indicated in Figure 7A, the BCG Grid is divided into four quadrants,
based on relative market growth and SBU shares. The grid is perhaps best
known for its clever labeling of each grid—stars, question marks, cash
cows, and dogs. Stars are SBUs that have good prospects—that is, relatively
high market shares and high rates of market growth. These are rapidly
growing units that require high investment. Uncertain SBUs—question
marks—are those that have low market shares but are located in rapidly
growing markets. These must be evaluated for whether the organization
should invest additional funds in them or should spin them off. Cash cows
are well-positioned SBUs (high market shares) that have limited prospects
for further growth (slow growth markets); thus, they become targets for
drawing off funds for use in building up the star and, as appropriate, question mark SBUs. Finally, dogs have low market shares and their markets
have low expected rates of growth. These SBUs represent possible cash
traps, in which significant continued investment is needed. Because they
have little hope for growth and return, dogs can become candidates to be
sold. Organizations thus seek a balance among these SBUs, in terms of having the ability to both shift funds across the quadrants and spread risk
across the SBUs.

Many problems exist in the use of the BCG Grid, the most significant of
which has to do with the appropriateness of using single indicators for each
of the two main dimensions. Is it reasonable to believe that market shares
fully capture the essence of strategic strength? Do market rates of growth
fully represent expected cash flows and profits? In fact, many other factors
can account for growth and strategic strength. Therefore, although this tool
is very popular and relatively easy to apply and use in assessment (high face
validity), it should be used in conjunction with other analytic tools.

Figure 7B. GE Business Screen

		High	Winner	Winner	Question Mark
Competitive Position		Medium	Winner	Average Producer	Loser
		Low	Profit Producer	Loser	Loser
			High	Medium	Low

Market Attractiveness

The GE Business Screen

The General Electric Company created an expanded version of the BCG Grid called the *GE Business Screen*. GE added a number of factors to the analysis of strategic position and industry or market attractiveness (Hoffer Schendel and Schendel 1978):

1. Market attractiveness
   • Market growth
   • Market size
   • Capital requirements
   • Competitive intensity

2. Competitive position
   • Market share
   • Technological know-how
   • Product quality
   • Service network
   • Price competitiveness
   • Operating costs

These factors were then weighted and summarized, and the results were broken into three ranks—high, medium, and low—per dimension (see Figure 7B). Because it is composed of multiple measures and possible weighting schemes, the GE Business Screen is less intuitive than is the BCG Grid, although it should provide a more valid basis for assessment.

Figure 7C. Mission-based Portfolio Matrix

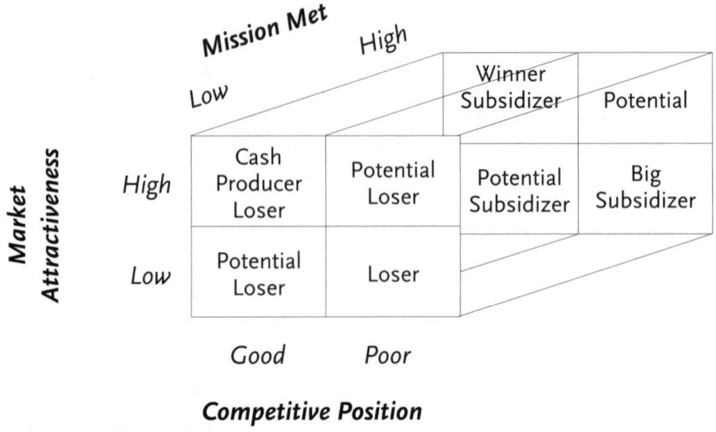

As with the BCG Grid, the GE Screen can provide rough guidance on which business units to keep and so on. Those labeled "winners" should be funded. The "profit producer," "average producer," and "question mark" should be held and watched for possible funding, cash drain, or divestment. Those labeled "losers" should be considered for divestment.

The Mission-Based Matrix

Neither of the above two matrixes considers the purposes of the organization, which can be an important limitation for healthcare organizations because of the importance of mission in this highly distinctive industry. Therefore, a useful modification of the GE Screen is the addition of a third dimension to the analysis: mission met. This is what is done in the mission-based matrix.

As can be seen in Figure 7C, the matrix assesses the extent to which the SBUs contribute to the organization's mission. Those that do not do well in this regard are classified as either "losers" or "potential losers," depending on the degree to which they meet the other two objectives in the analysis. They thus become strong candidates for divestment. The "cash producer loser" is likely reoriented, and efforts are made to bring it into compliance with the mission. "Winner subsidizers" are those businesses that support the organization's mission and generate significant cash flow to help subsidize business units that do support the mission.

Chapter 8

Horizontal Expansion

This [superiority of numbers] is in tactics, as well as in strategy, the most general principle of victory ....

—*Clausewitz (2000, 414)*

IN THIS CHAPTER, the power strategy that is most commonly pursued in all industries, including healthcare, is examined: *horizontal expansion.* Horizontal expansion is very important to strategy because it builds on and replicates existing strengths and bases for gaining competitive advantage. Simply, this strategy involves expansion in size within a single business arena. Horizontal expansion literally poured onto the healthcare landscape in the 1990s. At that time, nearly every healthcare organization seemed to either be participating in or contemplating acquisitions and mergers of other similar organizational combinations. This was especially true for the hospital sector: hospitals joined multihospital systems at an unprecedented rate in the 1990s.

This chapter focuses on horizontal expansion strategy for hospitals and hospital systems. Differences in how horizontal expansion is pursued by different hospital ownership types (e.g., not for profit, for profit, Catholic) are discussed. In addition, a critical distinction is shown to exist between company-level and local-market-level approaches to horizontal expansion. In many industries, horizontal strategy might be appropriately studied only at the company level. In healthcare, however, local horizontal strategy is a major source of competitive advantage because competition is intense and focused on territorial control at the local level. To help the reader understand some of the important variations in horizontal strategy, types of horizontal strategy are listed and examined in this chapter as well as their applications at both company and local levels.

OWNERSHIP TYPES

By the dawn of the 1990s, three different kinds of hospital ownership types had emerged: (1) not for profit, including public hospitals and church-related organizations; (2) Catholic; and (3) for profit. Ownership type might be considered an unusual basis for comparing strategic approaches, but the legal and tax status differences between hospital organizations are important determinants of organizational behavior in the hospital sector. Most especially, for-profit hospital organizations, motivated by the profit-maximizing expectations of their owners, are widely believed to be more efficient than other types of hospitals. Unfortunately, scant empirical evidence has been produced in support of this supposition, despite extensive research devoted to the topic (Gray 2000; Gray et al. 1999).

The 1990s, however, brought the differences between ownership types into stark relief, but not for the reasons previously thought to be important. The intense rivalry that erupted in that decade simply accentuated the distinctive approaches to horizontal strategy pursued by the three ownership types. That said, we examine horizontal strategy both pre- and post-1990 to see how horizontal strategy differed and, with time, changed for the three ownership types.

Pre-1990 Ownership and Horizontal Strategy

Before the 1990s, most for-profit organizations had pursued a kind of McDonald's strategy, investing in relatively small, easy to manage hospitals that were often located in small, uncontested markets or in high-growth suburban areas. This resulted in the formation of a number of very large, widely dispersed organizations such as HCA, Health Trust, Humana, National Medical Enterprises, American Medical International, and OrNda. Catholic hospital organizations, strongly driven by the mission-related objectives of their sponsors, also had become fairly large and widely dispersed. Like their for-profit counterparts, Catholic hospitals were often located in urban areas: 68 percent of Catholic hospitals were urban, while for profits and not for profits had 70 and 50 percent of their hospitals in urban markets, respectively.

The profiles of not-for-profit hospitals and systems thus differed strikingly from those of Catholics and for profits. By 1989, 79 percent of not-for-profit hospitals were not members of multihospital systems at all, compared to 16 and 18 percent, respectively, for Catholic and for-profit hospitals. This difference, however, did not mean that the not for profits were not involved in multihospital system formation. About 173 not-for-profit multihospital systems had formed by that time, compared to 76 Catholics and 46 for profits. A number of those systems were fairly prominent, such as Lutheran Health Systems, Adventist Health Systems, Alliant Health Systems, Intermountain Health Care, and Great Plains Health Alliance. On the other hand, the number of hospitals that most of these systems owned was small and most of their owned hospitals were tightly clustered within or around single markets, compared to the highly dispersed pattern typical for Catholics and for profits.

Because of their overwhelming numbers (representing nearly 72 percent of all acute care general hospitals), the not-for-profit hospitals (freestanding and in systems) held the key to the evolution of strategy throughout the 1990s. These hospitals thus became the primary acquisition and merger targets for most of the existing and forming systems, regardless of ownership type. Also, nearly three-quarters of the large (more than 400 beds) urban hospitals were not for profit. This is significant because many of these hospitals served as catalysts for the formation of local integrated systems.

Post-1990 Ownership and Horizontal Strategy

In the 1990s, Catholic and for-profit systems, being relatively large and widely dispersed, were assumed to be in the strongest positions to dominate the merger and acquisition craze. However, that assumption turned out to be false. Why is that? First, the numerous not-for-profit hospitals tended to prefer acquiring or being acquired by hospitals and systems that were both local and culturally and strategically "cousins" (of the same ownership type). Common ownership type and local interrelationships were critical determinants of the systems that hospitals chose to join. Second, many important systems formed out of the initiative of large, usually not-for-profit hospitals. These systems pursued horizontal expansion locally primarily to shore up local referral relationships, exert greater leverage on local contract negotiations with managed care companies, and increase local market power. All of this produced an explosion in system formation, especially among not-for-profit hospitals.

Table 8.1 highlights the significant system growth that occurred among not-for-profit hospitals in the 1990s. Between 1989 and 2001, the numbers of for-profit systems declined by 30 percent, and the numbers of Catholic

Table 8.1. Growth in Hospital System Membership Between 1989 and 2001, by Ownership Type

	1989			2001			% Change (1989–2001)		
	# of Systems	# of Hospitals in Systems		# of Systems	# of Hospitals in Systems		% of Systems	% of Hospitals in Systems	
		Overall Total	Urban Only		Overall Total	Urban Only		Overall Total	Urban Only
Not for Profit	173	802	472	295	1,358	962	71	69	104
For Profit	47	670	670	33	607	439	–30	–9	–10
Catholic	76	535	354	56	602	421	–26	13	19
Total	296	2,007	1,313	384	2,566	1,822	30	28	39

Note: From 1989 to 2001, the number of acute care general hospitals declined by about 8 percent.

systems declined by 26 percent; both of these trends reflect mostly the consolidations that occurred, resulting in a number of very large systems. Between the same time period, the number of hospitals (overall and urban) controlled by for profits declined; those owned by Catholics increased only slightly. By contrast, the number of not-for-profit systems increased by a startling 71 percent. More importantly, the number of hospitals joining not-for-profit systems increased overall by 69 percent, and the number of urban hospitals joining such systems increased by 104 percent. During this period, most of the growth in not-for-profit systems occurred in and around individual local markets or was the result of regional expansion by some systems.

Despite the clear edge in absolute power enjoyed by Catholic and for-profit multihospital systems, in that period the need to gain relative power appeared to be the dominant strategic imperative for hospital system formation and growth. The not-for-profit hospitals and systems were simply in the best position to take the lead.

Some of the most sensational combinations of systems in that period, however, occurred among for-profit and Catholic systems, including the following:

• the merging of Columbia, HCA, HealthTrust, and Humana to form Columbia/HCA;
• the combination of National Medical Enterprises, American Medical International, and OrNda to form Tenet; and
• the joining of a number of Catholic order–sponsored systems into still larger Catholic systems such as Ascension, Catholic Healthcare West, and Bon Secours.

These formations are reflected in Table 8.2, which shows that the average size of for-profit and Catholic systems grew by 30 and 50 percent, respectively, while the average size of not-for-profit systems remained constant. Although the not for profits grew in terms of the numbers of hospitals joining their systems (see Table 8.1), their average system sizes were unchanged.

In addition to pursuing absolute size growth, the for-profit and Catholic multihospital systems also attempted to build strong local positions (relative power) in the 1990s. Columbia/HCA, for example, gave considerable priority to local market concentration in addition to emphasizing its highly touted (and, ultimately, failed) national expansion strategy.

Table 8.2. Growth in System Size Between 1989 and 2001, by Ownership Type

	Average Number of Hospitals per System		
	1989	2001	% Change
Not for Profit	4.6	4.6	0.0
For Profit	14.2	18.4	30.0
Catholic	7.0	10.8	50.0

LEVELS AND DIMENSIONS OF HORIZONTAL EXPANSION

The foregoing discussion highlights significant differences in the way horizontal expansion strategy has been used within the hospital sector. First, hospital systems have clearly pursued horizontal strategies at two levels: company and local market. Second, those strategies have varied depending on the sizes of the systems being produced and the geographic configurations that have resulted from system expansion.

The strategies used by HCA illustrate well the differences in horizontal strategy when pursued at company versus local levels. At the company level, HCA has over the years attempted to increase significantly its overall mass as an organization. At this level, decisions related to horizontal expansion tended to focus on such issues as achieving economies of scale and scope, determining the respective roles of corporate versus individual business units, deciding financial allocations and control, making leadership appointments, making decisions about market entry (or exit), and leveraging negotiations on medical/surgical supplies and pharmaceuticals. At the local level, HCA concentrated its horizontal expansion strategies on determining how local market advantages could be attained. For example, HCA's strong Denver cluster—HealthOne—has given considerable attention to the dynamics of competition that are typical of an oligopolistically structured market such as Denver. HCA is the lead player in that market, and it is locked in competitive battle with several strong local rivals, especially Centura Health, the number two player. HCA can therefore be expected to focus its local horizontal and other strategies on maintaining its dominant position in that market, which it has.

In local markets where it has strength, such as in Denver, HCA is likely to pursue a number of other market strategies related to its local horizontal strategy, including the following:

- Seeking opportunities for administrative coordination among its facilities
- Sharing in the management of the supply-distribution channel
- Promoting shared positions in the market
- Jointly recruiting clinical staff.

Furthermore, because HCA operates a large referral hospital in Denver—Presbyterian–St. Luke's—as well as a number of smaller community hospitals, it might be expected to pursue the advantages attributable to clinical differentiation and integration across its facilities.

By contrast, HCA might take a different approach in applying horizontal expansion strategy in those markets where it does not have clusters of hospitals or it has very limited market shares. In the Washington, DC, market, for example, HCA operates only one hospital in Reston, Virginia. Horizontal expansion in such cases might lead HCA to acquire other hospitals in the market to build new facilities in growing areas in the metropolitan statistical areas, or it might simply stick to a niched strategy in an area in which it already has an established position. In any case, the issues HCA might consider in its pursuit of horizontal expansion strategies will likely differ enormously between corporate and local, and local issues will differ from one market to the next depending mostly on the strength of the organization's positions in those markets.

For some organizations, strategies at the company and local market levels are essentially indistinguishable. This is especially true for systems that have facilities in only one market. For INOVA Health System, for example, a five-hospital system based in the northern Virginia side of the Washington, DC, market, company and local market strategies are effectively the same. Many single-market organizations entertain at times the possibility of expanding beyond their local markets. In fact, INOVA has occasionally contemplated the possibility of acquiring facilities south and west of DC, both in nearby markets and in markets across the state. Thus, to the extent that it contemplates expanding beyond its local boundaries, INOVA's company-level thinking about horizontal strategy diverges from how it views horizontal strategy locally in the DC area.

The Key Dimensions

The foregoing discussion highlights two dimensions that serve as the primary bases for differentiating horizontal expansion strategies in the hospital sector:

1. *Organizational size*
2. *Geographic configurations*

Figure 8.1 illustrates the relationships of these two dimensions to company and local market levels and to the types of power strategy.

The many advantages associated with size, whether relative or absolute, should be fairly clear (see Chapter 7); on the other hand, how geographic configurations contribute to competitive advantage might not be easily recognized because such advantages are often very subtle. Nevertheless, they are highly important in the hospital sector as well as in most other healthcare sectors. Discussion in this section thus focuses on types of geographic configuration.

One important subdimension of geographic configuration is the relative *dispersion* of a system's hospitals across a given area. A system's hospitals' closeness to each other or distance separating them determines the way a system will go about managing, controlling, and integrating its hospitals. This is true for dispersion at both company and local levels. Close geographic proximities open up possibilities for

- seeking market dominance,
- sharing services,
- pursuing specialization,
- eliminating redundancies in clinical capacities,
- facilitating clinical integration and coordination,
- developing technologically advanced information networks,
- sharing other administrative functions,
- negotiating from strength for local managed care contracts, and
- coordinating competition across facilities.

Few of these advantages are available to systems whose facilities are widely dispersed.

A second important subdimension of geographic configuration applies exclusively to local strategies: the presence, or the lack, of a *hierarchical* structure among a local system's hospitals. The hierarchical structure of a

Figure 8.1. Dimensions of Horizontal Expansion and Their Relationship with Power Strategies, at Company and Local Levels

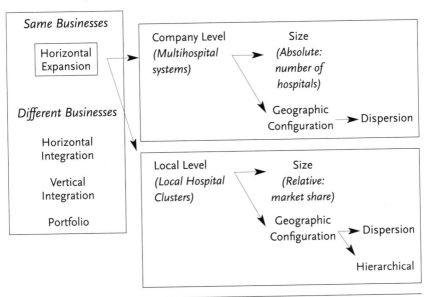

system relates to the degree to which hospitals in the local system differ functionally or by the particular role they each play within the system as a whole. One of the most important forms of internal system differentiation occurs when a system is composed of one or more large referral centers and a collection of smaller, more general community hospitals. Often referred to as a *hub-spoke model*, this unique structure offers the potential for complex tertiary and quaternary services to be provided by the hub and more general, primary and secondary services to be provided at the spokes, making the two hospitals functionally interdependent. This constitutes, in our terms, a hierarchically structured local-system model.

The possibility that such hierarchical arrangements can be created locally was the central idea underlying the integrated delivery system concept so widely advocated in the 1990s. In practice, the appearance of hierarchical structures does not necessarily mean that the systems have been successful in achieving workable interdependencies in practice. In fact, many hospital systems still appear to be on the high end of the learning curve in creating well-integrated delivery systems. Nevertheless, the 1990s produced a number of hub-spoke local systems, most of which were not for profit as would be expected given the preponderance of large hub hospitals in that ownership type. From a strategic perspective, these structural forms not only offer good prospects for functional integration; but, in many cases, they result in systems that dominate their local markets: the Carolinas HealthCare System cluster in Charlotte (47 percent share), Kaleida Health cluster in Buffalo (46 percent share), and Texas Health Resources cluster in Dallas (43 percent share).

The alternative to the hub-spoke model is a flatter configuration in which the hospitals are similar in size and complexity. In this configuration, the individual hospitals might differ more by the population segments served than by their clinical functionality or interdependencies. On the other hand, even the *flat model* configurations can achieve a degree of functional differentiation. Structurally similar facilities (similar sizes and mix of services), if located close together (low dispersion), are likely to experience high levels of service overlap. These facilities thus are prime candidates for administrative and service integration, and their services could be redistributed across their spatially proximate hospitals; over time, they could even evolve into more hierarchical arrangements. In recent years, many clustered hospitals have achieved varying degrees of clinical and administrative sharing and specialization as a result of their being geographically close to one another. Many have also reinforced the potential for such sharing by taking the extra step of merging, forming a single organizational entity where before two or more hospitals existed (even though they were owned by the same system). On the other hand, such similar hospitals, if separated by greater distances in their markets, might focus more on local market penetration and coordinated efforts to compete in the marketplace rather than on pursuing functional integration.

The two model types—hub-spoke (hierarchical) and flat (relatively equal in size and functionality—represent two different approaches to gaining competitive advantage at the local level. The relative spatial dispersion of a local system's hospitals also should affect how those hospitals interrelate operationally, clinically, and strategically.

A number of other industries exhibit very complex cluster interrelationships (Porter 1998). Some of these involve vertical arrangements between different businesses that buy and sell from each other; examples are clusters within the automotive, pharmaceutical, and biotechnology industries. Other complex relationships (most notably in the banking and airline industries) are similar to the situations for hospitals, where multiple units within the same businesses differ by their functional complexity and therefore the roles they play within their broader systems. Hospitals

Figure 8.2. Dispersion Patterns at Company Level, by Size

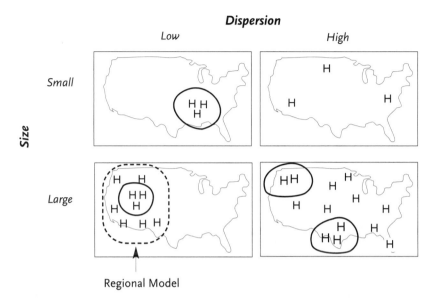

Local market clusters are two or more hospitals that are members of the same system and are in the same local market. Many of the small, low-dispersion multihospital systems are in single-market clusters.

are fairly unique, however, in that cluster differentiation and integration is primarily achievable only at the local level, which is especially true within the large- and medium-sized markets or between urban and nearby rural facilities.

GEOGRAPHIC CONFIGURATION AT THE COMPANY LEVEL

Differences in dispersion patterns exist among multihospital systems, large and small; such differences are illustrated in Figure 8.2. The small, tightly clustered systems tend to have facilities in only one market. On the other hand, the larger, tightly clustered systems often span multiple markets that are close together; we refer to this pattern as a *regional model*. By definition, the widely dispersed systems, large or small, are spread at considerable distances across multiple markets.

Catholic and for-profit hospital systems dominate the highly dispersed category, for both large and small systems; not-for-profit systems dominate the more tightly clustered types. Table 8.3 displays the percentage of systems in each of the three ownership types. These types are classified (as

Table 8.3. Dispersion Patterns at Company Level, by Ownership Type

		Dispersion Pattern for Systems (%)			
		Single Market[1]	Regional[2]	Dispersed[3]	Average Distance[4]
Ownership Type	Not for Profit	60	37	3	50
	For Profit	18	21	61	557
	Catholic	18	32	50	307

1. Single-market pattern is the multihospital system that is either in a single MSA or in only rural areas within a single state.
2. Regional pattern is the multihospital system that is in more than one market; the average distance between the system's hospitals and the system's geographic center is less than 150 miles.
3. Dispersed pattern is the multihospital system that is in more than one market; the average distance between the system's hospitals and the system's geographic center is 150 miles or greater.
4. Average distance is based on the distances between the corporate headquarters and each hospital in the system—that is, if the location can be identified; otherwise measurement is from the largest hospital located in the state that is in the approximate geographic center of the system.

of 2003) as either single market, regional, or highly dispersed systems. Sixty-one percent of the for-profit organizations are highly dispersed, compared to 50 percent of the Catholic systems and only 3 percent of the not for profits. The differences in dispersion by ownership type are significant.

Such differences are also reflected in the number of markets in which these systems have hospital facilities. The for-profit multihospital organizations were located in an average of 9.5 different markets, compared to averages of 5.5 markets for Catholic systems and 1.8 for not-for-profit systems. Among the large for-profit high-dispersion systems, HCA remained the most involved in multimarket horizontal expansion, owning hospitals in 80 different markets. Tenet was second with hospitals in 42 markets. In the Catholic group, Ascension Health and Catholic Health Initiatives (CHI) were neck and neck: Ascension had hospitals in 31 markets and CHI had hospitals in 28. On the not-for-profit side, Banner Health had hospitals in 17 markets (it is now attempting to sell off a number of those hospitals); two Adventist systems—Adventist Health System and Adventist Health West—had hospitals in 16 and 13 markets, respectively.

Two important medium-sized systems differ greatly by their relative degrees of dispersion: Sutter Health and Catholic Health East. Sutter, a

24-hospital system headquartered in Sacramento, California, is a good example of a regional model. Sutter has spread into ten markets, nine of
which are urban and one is a collective of the rural areas in Northern
California. The distance separating Sutter hospitals from the corporate
headquarters is about 71 miles. The Sutter network also offers a wide range
of services, from long-term care to outpatient services to physician practices. The business diversity within Sutter is likely the result of its having
a regionally clustered system—that is, its hospitals' close geographic proximities are highly compatible with integrative and comprehensive multiproduct strategies.

Catholic Health East (CHE), based in Newtown Square, Pennsylvania,
also has 24 acute care hospitals spread across ten markets. (It has four other
hospitals combined into the independently operated Baycare Health
System in Clearwater, Florida.) However, the system is more widely dispersed than is Sutter: CHE's hospitals spread from Maine to Florida, and
the distance between the hospitals and the headquarters is about 280 miles.
Given its high dispersion across markets, CHE corporate delegates relatively
high levels of authority to the local facilities. In fact, CHE is organized
around three regional health systems, each of which has a high degree of
autonomy in deciding how it will operate its regional cluster of hospitals
and other facilities. Sutter is also organized around geography; however,
because of the tight geographic proximities of its facilities, the system's
chief operating officer oversees coordination among its service areas. Thus,
Sutter and CHE not only differ significantly in their strategic configurations but also in their decision-making structures.

For an example of a multimarket horizontal expansion strategy pursued by a specialty hospital organization, see Strategy Note 8.1.

Geographic Expansion Strategies in Other Healthcare Sectors

Interestingly, managed care companies have increasingly moved toward
multimarket strategies, leading to high dispersion. Many Blue Cross plans,
for example, which were traditionally single-state organizations, have been
expanding rapidly across the country in response to changing market conditions. Many have even restructured themselves as for profits, a necessary first step for them to engage successfully in multimarket expansion.
As an example, Anthem Inc., a Blue Cross organization originally located
in Indiana, is now a for-profit, multimarket managed care company. It
has acquired Blue Cross plans in nine states, including Indiana, Ohio,
Kentucky, Kansas, Colorado, Nevada, Connecticut, New Hampshire, and

STRATEGY NOTE 8.1. MEDCATH: A SPECIALTY SYSTEM'S HORIZONTAL EXPANSION

MedCath, Inc., a for-profit system headquartered in Charlotte, North Carolina, owns ten heart hospitals (has three others under development) and runs a number of cardiac and related laboratories. To fortify its position as a quality provider, MedCath hired The Lewin Group to compare MedCath services to those of a large group of peer hospitals (i.e., general hospitals that provided cardiac services) across the country. The Lewin Group's findings showed that heart hospitals had a 12.1 percent lower in-hospital mortality rate for Medicare cases. Lengths of stays were also shorter (4.12 days versus 4.99 days). A much higher proportion of patients were also discharged to their homes rather than to other healthcare facilities (89.6 percent versus 72.4 percent (MedCath 2003).

MedCath represents a new breed of specialty systems that can challenge established community hospital providers. As such challenges make inroads, the established providers are beginning to react. In Indianapolis, Indiana, for example, a number of established players are planning heart hospitals in the hopes of saving costs, improving quality, and shoring up their positions in the cardiac business. In addition, three systems are constructing separate heart hospitals: Community Health Network (formally Community Hospital System), St. Vincent's Hospital, and St. Francis Hospital, all of which are located in Indianapolis, Indiana. Several of these organizations even advertise that their heart hospitals are going "digital," which will give doctors, at patients' bedside, instant Internet access to everything from medical records to menu preferences. The major system in Indianapolis, Clarian Health System, has created an internal heart hospital within its hospital space; that is, it has set aside an area within its existing facility and designated it as its heart hospital.

All of these specialized expansions represent the horizontal battles brewing within the specialty segment of the acute care hospital business.

Maine. In addition, Anthem has recently acquired Trigon Healthcare Inc., a Virginia-based, for-profit Blue Cross company; this acquisition brings Anthem's state representation up to ten. Such expansions are essential for Anthem, which hopes to benefit from larger scale and deeper pockets. (It expects to generate over $14 billion in annual revenues once the acquisition of Trigon is complete.) Also, the expansions will enable Anthem to make the much-needed investments in information system infrastructure, which is so essential to the managed care business. Gains in overall mass also should help Anthem to compete with the other important and rapidly expanding managed care companies as well as to countervail the growing market power of local provider systems.

Actually, managed care companies do not engage in local market horizontal strategies per se. This is because they operate as single entities in individual markets; therefore, location (let alone multiple locations locally) is not relevant to their strategies at the local level. Managed care companies focus locally on penetration, not acquisitions of multiple sites. For an example of how a vertically integrated managed care organization can engage in horizontal expansion strategies, see Strategy Note 8.2.

STRATEGY NOTE 8.2. KAISER: A VERTICALLY INTEGRATED ORGANIZATION'S HORIZONTAL EXPANSION

Horizontal expansion is most commonly associated with single-business enterprises, but complex, multibusiness organizations also engage in this strategy. For example, a vertically integrated organization, once it has refined its business practices, can replicate (horizontally) the vertical model in other markets. Kaiser is a good example of an organization that has done such a thing. In its first 30 years (1930s through 1950s), Kaiser perfected its vertical model in California, Washington, Oregon, and Hawaii. In its next 30 years, it expanded even further, establishing its model in eight additional states and Washington, DC. Although Kaiser did not transplant the complete vertical model (the hospital portion was not taken beyond California), it nevertheless built on its experience with vertical as it expanded horizontally.

Multimarket expansion has also been tried in the physician sector but with limited success, at least to date. In the 1990s, major physician practice management (PPM) companies attempted to expand across markets, hoping to become nationally dispersed systems. Following the hospital model, PhyCor and MedPartners, once the two largest PPMs, set out to expand nationwide as well as to build strong market positions locally. They even considered aligning at the local level with equally strong hospital systems, thereby creating highly powerful integrated delivery systems. By the end of the 1990s, the multimarket strategies for most PPMs failed. In 1997, PhyCor and MedPartners attempted to merge with each other, an effort that preceded their demise as companies by only a year or two: In 1998, Caremark, MedPartners's pharmacy benefits management division, completed the sell-off of MedPartners physician groups; PhyCor is now engaged in managing independent practice associations of physicians and provides consulting services to self-insured employers.

The above and other such examples raise serious questions about whether multimarket expansion strategies should be pursued within the physician sector. Single-market expansion strategies, by contrast, are very important for physician organizations. Many successful physician group practices have been established across the country and many have grown steadily. A number of physician-based organizations now run large, complex delivery systems as well, such as Mayo Clinic and The Cleveland Clinic. Both Mayo and The Cleveland Clinic have experimented with multimarket expansion. Mayo, a Rochester, Minnesota–based integrated system, has acquired facilities in surrounding nonurban areas and placed satellite facilities far away—in Jacksonville, Florida, and Scottsdale, Arizona. The Cleveland Clinic has pursued a similar strategy, acquiring a number of hospitals locally and establishing facilities in Fort Lauderdale and Naples, Florida. Note that the multimarket moves by Mayo Clinic and The Cleveland Clinic are the exception for not-for-profit physician-based systems.

Nonurban Organizational Types

Company-level horizontal strategies also differ significantly by whether or not the organizations concentrate on urban or on nonurban markets (or both). The structures of urban and nonurban markets differ greatly and, as a result, so do the corresponding horizontal strategies of the multihospital systems operating within those markets. Perhaps the most important difference between urban and nonurban markets is that rural competitors tend to stand alone within the small communities where they are located.

Interestingly, 37 percent of nonurban hospitals are members of multihospital systems, compared to 68 percent of urban hospitals. On the other hand, because of the small sizes of the nonurban markets, the hospitals or small clusters located in these communities exercise very high levels of monopoly power. Despite this, many nonurban markets are quite "contestable" (Baumol, Panzar, and Willig 1988). In fact, many competitors in nonurban markets must work very hard to counter threats emanating from rivals located in other nearby communities and urban markets, even if those rivals are located some distance away.

Many urban rivals can, and often do, draw patients away from their nonurban competitors, forcing the latter to be very strategic if they hope to survive (let alone remain independent) in the long run. This interdependency between urban and nonurban markets has produced interesting strategic organization types. The hospital systems that compete in nonurban markets differ dramatically by how they approach horizontal expansion—that is, by how they use size and geographic configuration to gain competitive advantage and how they structure urban and nonurban hospital and physician relationships.

One of the most important types of organization is the *urban-rural system*. The large, not-for-profit BJC health system, headquartered in Saint Louis, Missouri, is one example of an urban-rural organization. The BJC Barnes-Jewish Hospital, a St. Louis, Missouri, referral center, provides tertiary and quaternary services to BJC's regional network of hospitals and physicians located in both urban and nonurban areas in and around St. Louis. Typically, these urban-rural systems are relatively small, multimarket, and tightly clustered (low dispersion).

Another organizational type is the *rural-based system*. These systems typically join nonurban referral centers with smaller nonurban hospital and physician networks. Geisinger Health System, located in Danville, Pennsylvania (a nonurban community), is an example of a rural-based system. The Geisinger Medical Center, a 440-bed Level-I trauma and referral center, serves as the hub for this system. Geisinger has engaged in a variety of strategies to ensure that its referral facility maintains its referral base. In the 1990s, for example, it entered into a strategic alliance with the Penn State Milton S. Hershey Medical Center. If that alliance had succeeded, it would have eliminated (or brought under limited control) an important urban-based competitor for nonurban referrals. Geisinger also attempted other maneuvers to shore up its base. It acquired the Geisinger Wyoming Valley Medical Center in Wilkes-Barre, Pennsylvania, and built a network of around 60 Geisinger medical practices in the region. Also, Geisinger continued to build its not-for-profit rural HMO, which it had established in the early 1970s. That HMO now serves around 300,000 members in nearly 40 Pennsylvania counties, and it ties Geisinger to a large network of physicians and hospitals throughout the region. In other words, even though Geisinger is the sole provider in a nonurban community, it has aggressively applied horizontal (and some vertical) strategies to counter the erosion of its market by strong urban rivals. Rural-based systems tend to be small, multimarket, and tightly clustered.

A third organizational type builds on the advantages of pure mass rather than on local relationships: the large *multihospital system*. A number of very prominent examples of this particular type exist, including both for-profit and not-for-profit organizations. Four of the most recognized for-profit systems are Triad Hospitals, Inc.; Health Management Associates (HMA); Community Health Systems, Inc.; and LifePoint Hospitals, Inc; each of these owns between 22 and 55 hospitals. Community and LifePoint are almost exclusively nonurban, while HMA and Triad have around 60 percent of their hospitals in small urban areas. In effect, these four systems specialize in small markets and communities where they can be sole providers and thereby enjoy high market shares. These systems tend to be very large, multimarket, and highly dispersed, and they place little emphasis on interfacility integration or strategic coordination.

A variation on this type can be found in the not-for-profit sector. The Sioux Valley Health System of Sioux Falls, South Dakota, for example, runs around 30 hospitals located in Nebraska, Minnesota, Iowa, and South Dakota. Many such not-for-profit systems, however, tend to be highly regionalized. They are dispersed typically within a single state (e.g., the Iowa Health System) or within geographically proximate states (e.g., the Sioux Valley Health System). By comparison to the for-profit examples, these systems tend to focus more on intermarket and facility integration and coordination.

One final organization type is the *contract management company*. A number of urban hospital systems contract to manage various nearby, usually small, nonurban hospitals. Nearly all of these contract management companies are not-for-profit. The management business for them is closely tied to their need to shore up referral relationships. For them, geographic proximities are key to their involvement in nonurban markets.

Thus, except for these systems' tendency to rely on contractual relationships, they differ little from urban-rural systems. A couple of other organizations are primarily in the business of contract management. Quorum Health Resources, a 1980s spin-off of HCA, is the largest such company. It manages around 250 hospitals; some of these are urban but most are nonurban and nearly all are small. Over the past several decades, Quorum began buying hospitals to compliment its management business, resulting in 22 hospital acquisitions. In 1998, Triad acquired Quorum, primarily because it wanted to capture Quorum's owned facilities. After much deliberation, Triad decided to retain Quorum's management business, a decision that converted Triad into a horizontally integrated organization (which loosely integrates the operation of both owned and management businesses). Quorum itself is a large, for-profit, highly dispersed, multimarket organization that aggregates hospitals using contractual, rather than ownership, arrangements.

GEOGRAPHIC CONFIGURATION AT THE LOCAL LEVEL (URBAN)

Local urban clusters are distinguished using two key dimensions of geographic configuration: dispersion and hierarchical structure. Local clusters can be either single-market systems (e.g., INOVA in the DC area) or local combinations owned by multimarket systems (e.g., HCA's Denver cluster, HealthOne). Figure 8.3 displays geographic configuration dimensions at the local level. Two dispersion patterns are highlighted: (1) high dispersion and (2) low dispersion (hospitals cluster within a single sector of a market). The hierarchical dimension also divides into two types: (1) high hierarchical (hub-spoke) and (2) low hierarchical (flat or relatively equal sizes and capacities across the hospitals).

Figure 8.4 shows two clusters in the Chicago market demonstrating dispersion differences between hospital clusters. As shown in the figure, the hospitals owned by Advocate Health Care, a Chicago-based not-for-profit organization that operates nine acute care general hospitals in the market, are more widely dispersed than are those owned by Resurrection Health Care, a Chicago-based eight-hospital Catholic company. Advocate is the product of a merger in 1995 between the Evangelical Health System and the Lutheran General Health System; by chance, this merger resulted in a fairly dispersed pattern of coverage across the Chicago market. Resurrection came into being when the hospitals sponsored by the Sisters of the Holy Family of Nazareth and the Sisters of the Resurrection merged.

Figure 8.3. Geographic Configuration Patterns at Local Level

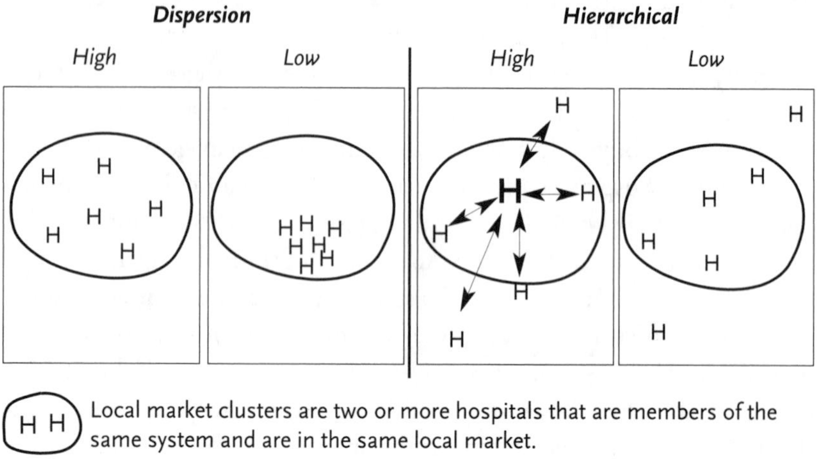

| | Dispersion | | Hierarchical | |
| High | Low | | High | Low |

Local market clusters are two or more hospitals that are members of the same system and are in the same local market.

Notes:
1. Single-market urban systems are also defined as local market clusters.
2. Many multimarket systems have one or more clusters within them.
3. Clusters are defined and measured for urban MSAS only.

This merger produced a more compact model, again by chance. Given its more general coverage of the Chicago market, Advocate should be better positioned to function as a full market provider. Resurrection, because of its more compact configuration, should gain advantages from its relative dominance over a smaller geographic sector within the market. The close proximities between Resurrection's hospitals also should open the door wider, than perhaps for Advocate, for its hospitals to engage in the sharing, consolidation, and redistribution of clinical services.

Numerous examples exist of local hospital combinations that have great potential to integrate hierarchically among their members. An ideal example is the Orlando Regional Healthcare System in Orlando, Florida. At the functional and geographic center of this system (see Figure 8.5) is the Orlando Regional Medical Center. This 517-bed referral center has all of the bells and whistles of a major tertiary care center. It is a teaching and research institution that offers a Level I trauma center; airborne emergency transport; sophisticated burn and tissue rehabilitation services; and a wide variety of advanced diagnostic and laboratory testing, medical, and other services. In addition, the system includes seven community general hospitals, a cancer center, and a women's and children's hospital. As shown

Figure 8.4. Dispersion Patterns for Two Major Single-Market, Multihospital Systems in the Chicago Metropolitan Area

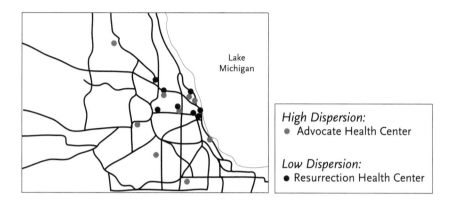

Lake Michigan

High Dispersion:
● Advocate Health Center

Low Dispersion:
● Resurrection Health Center

in the figure, these facilities are dispersed throughout the Orlando area, and the medical center, located at the geographic center of the cluster, serves as a functional fulcrum or hub for the system as a whole. For a discussion of whether this hierarchical strategy is a variation of horizontal expansion or vertical integration, see Strategy Note 8.3.

Nearly all large, complex hospitals have the potential of being organized within a hierarchical configuration; many have done so, resulting in various horizontal equivalents to the Orlando Regional system. Some of the most important of these are major teaching and research institutions. One such system is the Memorial Hermann Healthcare System (MHHS) in Houston, Texas. MHHS is large and represents a strategic response expected from a major academic medical center that competes directly with other such centers in the same market area (in this case, it competes with two other such centers that are right next door). MHHS is the product of a 1997 merger between the internationally recognized Hermann Hospital (located in the Texas Medical Center—see Strategy Note 8.4) and the community-based Memorial Health System. The merger immediately produced a market leader that now controls around 25 percent of the Houston market. As with Orlando Regional, MHHS serves as the hub and its community hospitals serve as the spokes. Prior to the merger, Memorial was conspicuous for having pursued an unabashed dispersion strategy within the local market; it even named its individual hospitals for the particular geographic sector they were intended to serve—that is,

Figure 8.5. Orlando Regional Healthcare System: A Hierarchically Configured, Highly Dispersed Organization

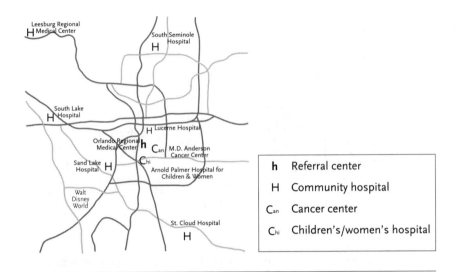

Memorial Northwest, Memorial Southeast, and so on. The addition of Hermann added the centerpiece needed for Memorial to move toward a more clinically configured hierarchical model.

As MHHS grew in size and market power, it began to venture outside of the Houston market. It has, for example, acquired three hospitals in the Beaumont–Port Arthur, Texas, market, which is located a little over 60 miles from Houston. The Beaumont acquisitions, therefore, complement the hierarchical model (now evolving into a regional model) already developed within the Houston market.

Table 8.4 shows that the geographic patterns of local clusters differ across the three ownership types. In this table, the range in patient days between the largest and smallest hospital cluster is used to indicate the possibility of a hierarchical (hub-spoke) configuration. As can be seen in the table, the not-for-profit clusters have a higher average range in patient days between the smallest and largest facilities in each cluster, and the for-profit systems have the lowest. This indicates a relatively greater prospect for the not for profits to evolve to the hierarchical configuration, relative to the for-profit clusters. The for-profit clusters, on the other hand, have the highest average distances between their locally clustered hospitals—8.5 miles—whereas the not-for-profit clusters are more tightly

STRATEGY NOTE 8.3. IS HIERARCHICAL CONFIGURATION HORIZONTAL OR VERTICAL?

Given the many and often complex interrelationships within functionally integrated and differentiated systems, it is tempting to conclude that the hierarchically structured hospital combinations represent mere variations of vertical integration. However, the presence or possibility of interorganizational flows of patients, services, and information need not mean that vertical arrangements exist. Virtually any production activity involves production flows of one kind or another. Lab tests, x-ray exams, clinical consults, and other clinical procedures move within and between provider units everyday. The hierarchical model simply structures those production activities a little differently than might be the case if the services were more generally intermixed within individual facilities.

Perhaps this distinction between vertical and the hierarchical version of horizontal expansion is only a matter of degree. If the provider units, say, were differentiated by specialty—that is, if they each represented distinctly different businesses such as acute care, rehabilitation, and psychiatric—then the alignment of such units might constitute more of a vertical or buyer-seller relationship. Functional differentiation among hospital members within the same general business (say, acute care), however, tends to fall short of exclusivity or full specialization. Although the individual hospitals might assume some specialized functions (one a referral center and the others community hospitals), they all by definition still engage in general acute care. Given the preponderance of functions that are common among them, such system arrangements should appropriately be characterized as horizontal expansion.

In the end, the distinctions being drawn here are not critical. The key ideas are differentiation, integration, and their impacts on competitive advantage. These concepts apply to all power strategy models, regardless of the labels we place on them.

STRATEGY NOTE 8.4. THE TEXAS MEDICAL CENTER

The Texas Medical Center (TMC) is located in Houston, Texas. TMC is not a provider; it is quite possibly the largest single-campus conglomeration of medical institutions in the world, including more than 40 provider institutions, two medical schools, and four schools of nursing. It houses the Shriners Hospital for Children and the M. D. Anderson Cancer Center as well as three large, internationally renowned, private general acute care hospitals: The Methodist Hospital, St. Luke's Episcopal Hospital, and Memorial Hermann Hospital.

The conglomeration of rivals within the TMC campus has produced some fascinating competitive dynamics over the years. The three major referral centers have made various attempts to merge with one another. In the 1990s, Methodist and St. Luke's, for example, attempted to merge, an effort that failed to materialize. St. Luke's then attempted a new strategy. It tried to link up with Columbia/HCA's local cluster of community hospitals. This too failed, having been rebuffed by a court challenge initiated by the TMC itself. Of course, had this merger succeeded, St. Luke's would have served as the primary referral center for the HCA community hospitals.

compacted locally, with 6.7 miles on average. Finally, the not-for-profit clusters enjoy the highest average shares (unadjusted for market size), with 31 percent. These numbers tell an important story about local clustering. Relative to Catholic and for-profit clusters, the not-for-profit clusters appear to be better positioned not only to become hierarchical, but also to dominate their local markets in terms of market shares.

HCA'S HORIZONTAL EXPANSION STRATEGIES

The case of HCA illustrates how horizontal expansion strategies can and do evolve over time. Looking at HCA also allows us to compare horizontal strategy pursued at both company and local levels within the same system.

HCA has passed through tumultuous periods of change in recent decades. It has engaged in aggressive horizontal expansion strategies and

Table 8.4. Geographic Configuration for Local (Urban) Clusters, by Ownership Type

		Dispersion	Hierarchical	
	# of Clusters[1]	Average Distance[2]	Average Range in Patient Days[3]	Average Market Shares
Not for Profit	256	6.7	91,317	31%
For Profit	88	8.5	44,602	21%
Catholic	102	7.8	64,572	30%

1. A cluster is defined as two or more hospitals in the same system and in the same market.
2. Average distance is measured between the largest hospital in the cluster and the other hospitals in that cluster.
3. Average range of patient days is based on the differences in patient days between the largest and the smallest hospitals in the cluster.

has had to adapt organizationally in the face of new strategic opportunities, market threats, and legal challenges. Figure 8.6 displays HCA's shifting horizontal pattern (company level) over the past several decades. The 1980s began with three major, and at that time, for-profit, companies: HCA, Humana, and Columbia. In that decade, in an attempt to pare down to basics and develop a more manageable system, HCA spun off HealthTrust, forming the third largest multihospital system in the country; it also spun off Quorum Health Resources, the hospital management company, which, effectively, was a different business. In 1984, Humana, then the second largest multihospital system, created an HMO product called Humana Health Care Plans, which grew into a major managed care player (see Chapter 9). However, in 1993, Humana spun off its hospital business, which became Galen, and that was acquired by a much smaller, relatively unknown Texas-based organization called Columbia. In 1994, Columbia then acquired HCA and HealthTrust in succession and renamed itself Columbia/HCA. In effect, Columbia swallowed up within about a year's time the three largest multihospital organizations in the country, creating a $21-billion-dollar-a-year, 250-hospital multibusiness company.

From there, Columbia/HCA entered a period of continued growth and legal challenge. In 1999, it spun off two companies—Triad and LifePoint—and changed its name back to HCA. As if to complete the cycle of acquisitions and spin-offs, Triad acquired Quorum in 2001, resulting

Figure 8.6. Evolution of HCA: Changing Horizontal Expansion Strategies at the Company Level

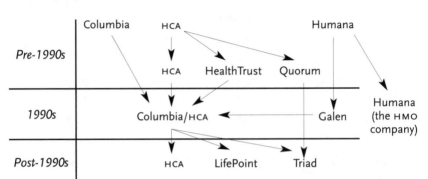

once again in three major multihospital companies reformulated out of the original three. Today, HCA remains large, multimarket, and highly dispersed, although it passed through a rather circuitous route to get there. Table 8.5 summarizes HCA's changing horizontal strategies in terms of geographic configuration dimensions at both company and local levels. In the early years, HCA engaged in a steady strategy of growth, targeting business-friendly states and high-growth locations. This resulted in an organization that owned or managed over 450 hospitals in the 1980s. At that time, HCA did not seek to cover the whole of the United States, choosing instead to concentrate its efforts on the southern and western parts of the country. HCA's company-level dispersion pattern was high before the 1990s.

Before the 1990s, HCA appeared to emphasize the acquisition of hospitals located in rapid growth sectors within individual markets. It did not emphasize large, center-city hospitals, although it tried to acquire some of these from time to time, but with little success. In markets in which HCA ended up with more than one hospital, the dispersion pattern tended to be fairly spread out, which can be characterized as moderate dispersion at the local level at that time. HCA also placed very little emphasis on hierarchical hub-spoke arrangements or on clinical integration. Rather, it stressed efficient management of individual hospitals overall, as opposed to their integration locally.

The mid-1990s produced a significant change in HCA's horizontal strategies. First, Columbia/HCA clearly pursued a national strategy, hoping to position itself to capture the multimarket managed care contracts of managed care organizations or contracted out by large *Fortune* 500

Table 8.5. HCA's Shifting Geographic Configuration, at Company and Local Levels

	Pre-1990s HCA	1990s Columbia/HCA	Post-1990s HCA
Company Level			
Dispersion	High	Very High	High
Local Level			
Dispersion	Moderate	High	Moderate
Hierarchical	Low	Moderate	Moderate

companies. Second, HCA bought fully into the prevailing logic that hospital systems had to dominate and be dispersed throughout their local markets, particularly if they hoped to capture managed care contracts locally. These ideas led to its emphasis on high dispersion, both nationally and locally. By pursuing multiple hospitals spread throughout a market, HCA hoped to offer comprehensive and geographically dispersed services to managed care companies. Also, HCA was no different from other hospital organizations in believing that integration would eventually produce improvements in quality, lower costs, and create better prospects for capturing managed care contracts. However, lacking hub hospitals in many markets (which it attempted mostly unsuccessfully to acquire in that period), HCA was unable to give significant priority to hierarchical arrangements. In sum, HCA's 1990s company-level dispersion strategies were very high (the national focus) and its local dispersion strategy was high. HCA's efforts to achieve hierarchical arrangements increased from low before the 1990s; because of the difficulty HCA encountered in accomplishing this model, its hierarchical strategy can be characterizes as moderate in the 1990s.

As HCA moved into the 2000s, shouldering the burden of a major legal challenge from the federal government (settled in 2002) and the disappointment of a failed national expansion strategy, it became a very different organization, not only culturally and structurally but strategically as well. It put in place new leadership and a new set of values and spun off a number of its hospitals, while grappling with continuing legal challenges. It dropped the name of Columbia, becoming once again HCA (a change in positioning strategy). Most especially, its horizontal strategy shifted once again. It pared back considerably its failed national expansion strategy, returning to its original emphasis on the southern and western regions of the country. All these efforts moved HCA back to high on the company-level dispersion strategy.

In addition, HCA now places somewhat less emphasis on covering all sectors of the local markets, recognizing that such played only a minor role in managed care contracting. HCA does retain its 1990's emphasis on market dominance, however; its selection of hospitals to spin off to Triad and LifePoint reflects an emphasis on maintaining local market concentration. Further, it chose to concentrate on those urban markets in which it already had strong market positions (or the possibility of gaining such), and it emphasized large markets to the extent possible.

Finally, HCA still gives priority to integration at the local market level, but now its focus is more on achieving administrative, rather than clinical, efficiencies. HCA's emphasis on hierarchical structures dissipated, with the exception of markets in which it has large hub hospitals. Strategies that the organization pursued for its local cluster in Richmond, Virginia, illustrate HCA's approach of integrating within a market in which it has a strong position. The two Richmond hospitals that HCA merged—Johnston Willis and Chippenham hospitals—happen to be geographically clustered on the south side of the James River. These two facilities remain as acute care hospitals, but they share services, name, and management structure. All of HCA's hospitals in the area attempt to coordinate supply distribution, planning for IT, and other management and service functions. Aside from efforts to rationalize clinical services across its two geographically proximate facilities, HCA is looking for opportunities to rationalize services among its remaining hospitals on the north side of the river. Successful clinical integration (hierarchical) across its local hospitals, however, still lags, although some hub-like distinctions are emerging among its hospitals.

CONCLUSION

This chapter addresses the strategy—horizontal expansion—that is not only the most important among power strategies but also among all other strategies; this is true for a number of reasons. First, horizontal expansion has the potential of altering dramatically the balance in competitive advantage locally, regionally, and nationally. Second, it (or any of the power strategies) is a costly strategy and thus deserves considerable organizational commitment if pursued.

The aggressive experimentation with horizontal expansion in the 1990s challenged very powerful, deeply imbedded institutionalized sources of power in individual organizations and markets specifically and in the healthcare industry generally. This aggressive application of power strategies can easily increase in intensity in the not-too-distant future. The industry is currently consummating the many changes that occurred in the 1990s, which is one reason why the merger and acquisition pace has dropped off considerably. However, market threats will likely intensify once again, further motivating many healthcare organizations to reenter the arena of horizontal expansion strategy. For example, inflation has picked up in the industry, and the need to manage the demand of aging baby boomers looms large. Further, a great, perhaps even increasing, need is evident for hospitals and systems to keep up with rapid changes in information technology and other advancements; capital is obviously needed to fund these investments. Hospital (and other provider) consolidation might be the only means by which such capital can be generated in the future.

If these and such trends occur, expansion strategies certainly will differ significantly from those in the 1990s. Today, the industry (at least the hospital sector) has a solid base on which to build, especially at the local level, their consolidation strategies. Future consolidation might focus on building regional systems and absolute power overall. Given the complexity, costliness, strategic importance, and probable renewed emphasis on power as a source of advantage, healthcare strategy analysts must gain a clear understanding of the many issues and models that are associated with horizontal expansion.

REFERENCES

Baumol, W. J., J. C. Panzar, and R. D. Willig. 1988. *Contestable Markets and the Theory of Industry Structure*, revised ed. San Diego, CA: Harcourt Brace Jovanovich.

Clausewitz, K. V. 2000. "Superiority in Numbers." In *The Book of War*, edited by C. Carr, 414. New York: Modern Library.

Gray, B. H., G. Carrino, S. Collins, and M. Gusmano. 1999. *The Empirical Literature Comparing For-Profit and Nonprofit Hospitals, Managed Care Organizations, and Nursing Homes: Updating the Institute of Medicine Study*. Washington, DC: Coalition for Nonprofit Healthcare.

Gray, B. H. 2000. "The Evolution of Investor-Owned Hospital Companies." *Perspectives in Medical Sociology*, 3rd ed., edited by P. Brown. Prospect Heights, IL: Waveland Press.

MedCath. 2003. [Online information; retrieved 1/03.] http://www.medcath.com.

Porter, M. E. 1998. *On Competition*. Boston: Harvard Business School Press.

Chapter 9

Vertical Integration

An army gathered together for a campaign was comparable to a town: it had a dense population and did not produce its own provisions. But, unlike a town, it has neither a preexisting transportation network nor any established pattern of local suppliers....

—Jones (1987, 46)

All armies—ancient and modern—have had to manage supply and distribution if they hoped to be victorious in war. A large army cannot survive long on the battlefield without sufficient food and supplies to sustain its fighting force. Thus, as Jones implies in the above quote, management and the structuring of the vertical supply channel often presented very serious challenges for invading armies. Armies that succeeded in overcoming major logistical problems, however, experienced considerable gains in military advantage.

The management of the vertical structure has also been a major concern in the healthcare industry. In fact, in the 1990s, many observers thought that the healthcare industry would move into a significant period of restructuring, focused primarily on integrating up and down the vertical channel (Conrad and Dowling 1990; Mick and Conrad 1988; Conrad and Shortell 1996; Enthoven 1980). This is because in healthcare the interrelationships among payment, delivery, supplies, and logistical support functions are so numerous, diverse, and highly complicated. Thus, by nearly any standard of performance, vertical integration appeared to be the logical structural response for improving communication, coordination, control, efficiencies, quality, satisfaction, access, and many other management and logistical problems in the industry. In a very specific sense, vertical integration was seen as a good way to manage the relationships between physicians and hospitals, relationships that historically have been so extensive and disorganized. Of course, vertical integration was also seen as a way to build up power in the marketplace.

HMOs, the *sine qua non* of vertical and, from the provider standpoint, the integrated delivery system, were thus viewed as efficient models for organizing healthcare and for aligning incentives for delivery. Ironically, despite its perceived importance, organized medicine has for years viewed vertical models as anathema to traditional approaches to delivering services. For this and other reasons, vertical integration should be recognized as carrying with it a significant overlay of normative sanctioning, punctuated by an extended history of provider antipathy.

In the 1990s, the environmental and market forces seemed fully aligned to facilitate a shift toward more vertical models. Most importantly, the growing power of managed care seemed primed to ignite a major restructuring focused on vertical. As we now know, however, vertical integration just did not take hold. Despite this, the experiment with vertical taught us much about the many limitations inherent in this unique approach to strategy, especially as applied to healthcare provider organizations. Given the many barriers that restrain the implementation of vertical, therefore, this chapter focuses mostly on the rationale for and the constraints that inhibit this important organizational model.

VERTICAL INTEGRATION BASICS

The strategy analyst would be wise to remember that despite its problems, vertical remains a major prospective strategic (and policy) approach for restructuring the healthcare industry. The healthcare environment can easily change once again, reestablishing conditions favorable to the formulation of vertical models. For this and many other reasons, the strategic analyst needs to understand how vertical might and might not contribute to competitive advantage in healthcare.

Supporting Arguments

Aside from many policy considerations, a number of strong strategic arguments support vertical integration. Mick (1990) classified these arguments in two conceptual arenas: (1) transaction-cost economics (Williamson 1975, 1986; Ouchi 1977) and (2) a strategic management perspective (Harrigan 1983; Porter 1985).

The *transaction cost* perspective is grounded on an efficiency argument: vertical integration is justified when the net costs of conducting transactions between buyers and sellers exceed the net benefits of relying on unstructured, negotiated transactions. Transaction costs are incurred when undertaking market exchanges, whether to obtain inputs or to dispose of outputs. These costs are not the same as the direct costs of production because transaction costs include the expenditures for monitoring, negotiating, and enforcing market exchanges. Mick summarized the transaction-costs argument using a diagram similar to that reproduced in Figure 9.1. A number of factors are associated with increased costs of market exchange, including the following, as indicated in the figure:

- uncertainty and complexity,
- bounded rationality,
- small-numbers bargaining,
- opportunism, and
- information impactedness.

The benefits associated with choosing to produce goods or services internally (in a vertical arrangement) appear on the right of the figure; they are as follows:

- goal congruence,
- control of processes,
- sequential decision making,
- conflict resolution, and
- adjustments to markets.

Uncertainty and complexity in market exchange, possibly the most frequently cited reasons for moving to vertical integration, increase the difficulties inherent in coordinating, sequencing, and controlling production. They also constrain the ability of managers to be rational about market decision making (bounded rationality). The existence of small numbers of buyers or sellers further complicates market exchange, given the added threat that powerful rivals bring to strategic choice. Consolidated market structures also provide a fertile environment for opportunistic behaviors (e,g., misrepresentation of intent within the market), thereby making predicting and controlling both prices and quality

Figure 9.1. Transaction-Cost Argument

Factors that Affect
Increased Costs

Benefits of Internal
Coordination

Uncertainty and Complexity

Bounded Rationality

Small-Numbers Bargaining

Opportunism

Information Impactedness

Vertical Integration

Goal Congruence

Control of Processes

Sequential Decision Making

Conflict Resolution

Adjustments to Markets

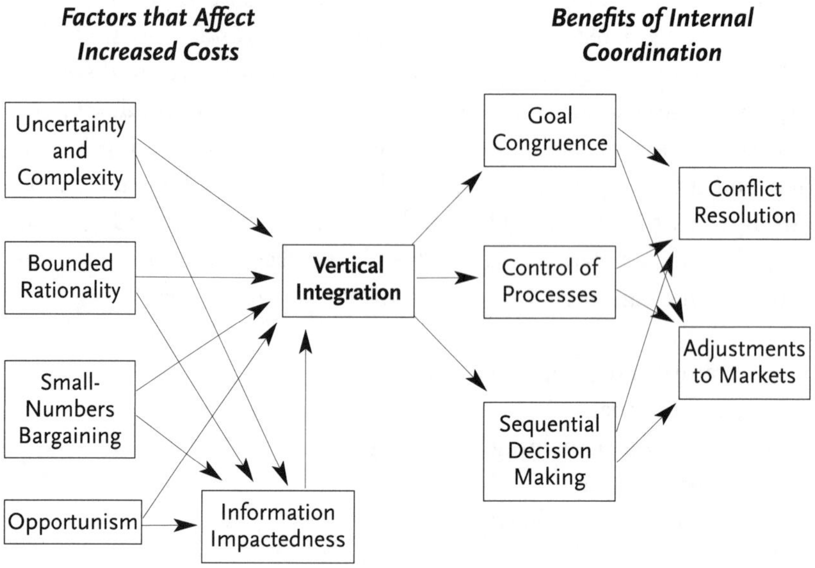

Source: Adapted from *Innovations in Health Care Delivery: Insights for Organization Theory*, edited by S. Mick. Copyright © 1990. This material is used by permission of John Wiley & Sons, Inc.

difficult for managers. All of the above challenge competitors to ensure that their market exchanges are conducted efficiently and that the outcomes of exchange meet their expectations. All such conditions open the door to vertical integration.

The *strategic management perspective* focuses more directly on general competitive advantage. In this respect, the transaction cost argument is subsumed under the strategic to the extent that gains in the efficiency of transactions contribute to competitive advantage. Porter (1980) identified a number of strategic arguments for and against vertical integration; a modified list of his arguments appears in Table 9.1. (In the table, the arguments are arranged within the five sources of competitive advantage.) All of the reasons listed in the table are important to healthcare organizations, although some have been especially important in recent years. Hospitals in the 1990s, for example, looked to vertical as a way to offset the growing complexity and threat of exchanges with managed care companies.

Table 9.1. Benefits and Costs of Vertical Integration

Benefits	Costs
Power	*Power*
• Increases organizational mass	• Raised height of exit barriers
• Offsets bargaining power and price distortions	*Performance*
• Elevates entry and mobility barriers	• Costs of overcoming mobility barriers
Positioning	• Increased operating lever-age and fixed costs
• Improves ability to differentiate the product	• Higher capital-investment requirements
Performance	• Balance in production capacities
• Captures economies of integrations by	• Differing managerial requirements; thus, greater costs of coordina-tion, compromise, and control
a. gaining economies of combined opera-tions	
b. achieving better internal control and coordination	
c. improving information exchange	• Dull incentives
d. avoiding the market	*Potential*
e. stabilizing relationships	• Foreclosed access to suppliers
• Enters a higher return business	
Potential	
• Taps into technology	
• Ensures supply or demand	
• Improves access to distribution channels and market information	*Pace*
Pace	• Reduced flexibility to change partners
• Defends against foreclosure	

Source: Concepts from Porter, M. E. 1980. *Competitive Strategy*. New York: The Free Press.

Provider Involvement

Many providers saw vertical as a vehicle for better positioning themselves in their markets. Intermountain Health Care (IHC), the Salt Lake City–based multihospital organization, has used the vertical strategy effectively to change and enhance its market image. Having entered the HMO business in 1983 and having acquired physician practices in the 1990s, IHC now describes itself on its web site almost as if it were a managed care, rather than a hospital, company: "Today IHC is a full-service, vertically integrated health care organization, where doctors, hospitals, and health plans work together in a mutual search for higher quality care and service." Also on their web site, the IHC logo includes the tag line, "Doctors, hospitals and health plans working together for you." IHC clearly sees value in touting its vertically integrated structure as a basis for gaining competitive advantage in its markets. The various businesses owned by IHC are also highly reinforcing. The HMO beneficiaries have access to IHC hospitals and physicians throughout the state, and the reputation of the IHC hospitals and doctors gives market value to IHC's HMO. IHC has also been a leader in information technology development, which should provide additional cost savings and system integration benefits across the system.

Perceiving in the 1990s that the costs of conducting exchanges with the increasingly powerful and aggressive managed care companies justified forward integration (i.e., integration downstream, toward the consumer), many hospitals considered following the lead of IHC and a select few other vertically integrated models, such as Kaiser Health Plan, by developing or acquiring their own HMO businesses or by sponsoring PPOs. However, few were successful in doing this. Aventis (2001) reported that by the beginning of 2000, only about 80 hospitals and a little more than 100 integrated systems owned HMOs. These numbers suggest that, at best, only about 2 percent of the acute care hospitals nationwide are involved in this important form of vertical integration. Nevertheless, IHC's apparent success (as well as continued success of a select few others), although fairly atypical, holds out the hope for many provider systems that vertical integration might in time become an important source of competitive advantage.

LIMITATIONS

Downstream vertical integration by hospitals (acquiring managed care businesses) seems a fairly natural strategic move. Besides the reasons given above, exchanges between providers and managed care companies are frequent and complicated by vigorous price negotiations, information complexity, referral approvals, and utilization and quality reviews. The information exchange and controls are managed within a complex web of information systems and bureaucracy, which create powerful switching costs that limit the degree to which contracts can be altered or moved from one provider to the next (or one managed care company to the next).

Vertical integration initiated by providers, in all of its forms, thus seems a logical next step in strategic evolution. So why has vertical not taken hold in the hospital industry? Some significant limitations constrain the pursuit of vertical integration as a power strategy for healthcare providers; three are especially important:

1. Lack of strategic fit
2. Competing with customers
3. Confounded strategic interrelationships

Of course, many other issues are associated with vertical integration, as Strategy Note 9.1 illustrates.

Lack of Strategic Fit

The first strategic problem limiting the hospital's forward integration into managed care (or backward integration by managed care) is a lack of congruence between the markets and the strategic and marketing objectives of the two businesses. Provider services are primarily delivered locally, while managed care markets tend to be much more expansive geographically, often reaching into many different markets. Thus, managed care companies need considerable flexibility to expand geographically, depending on shifts in demand and competition. By contrast, provider systems tend to be highly restricted to given markets, given the need for desirable locations, facilities, referral arrangements, clinical support services, local managed care contractual arrangements, and so forth. Also, entering provider markets by expanding capacity is difficult. Thus, multimarket expansion requires provider organizations to engage in mergers and acquisitions, which carries its own complications.

Managed care companies, by contrast, need mostly to establish marketing capitalization capacities if they decide to enter new markets. Vertical integration by a managed care company with a local provider system might therefore unduly tie the managed care company's hands in terms of geographic movement, strategic flexibility, and competition. Also, managed care products often need very large numbers of beneficiaries for them to be successful. This means that managed care companies will tend to contract with many buyers as well as with many local providers, many of which will be direct rivals to the provider systems with which they are vertically integrated. Providers, on the other hand, need to deeply penetrate their own geographic territories. Their HMO partners will not likely have achieved sufficient penetration of those areas to be capable of directing to them the levels of patients needed for the provider's survival.

Thus, these providers inevitably will have to contract with the direct rivals of their managed care partners. As a result of such misalignments of strategic objectives, relationships between vertically integrated managed care and provider companies are often compromised.

A number of prominent examples exist that show successful integrations of provider and managed care businesses. These include IHC (discussed above) as well as Spectrum Health in Grand Rapids, Michigan, and Sentara Healthcare in Norfolk, Virginia. Sentara, historically a single-market multihospital organization, forward integrated into the managed care business in 1984, having established Optima Health Plan. Ten years later, Sentara created a Medicaid HMO as well. Sentara's HMO businesses have, for the most part, covered the same area as that served by its hospitals, physicians, and other healthcare product lines. In time, the health plans expanded beyond the Norfolk market to other parts of southeastern Virginia and northeastern North Carolina. With further growth, Sentara's health plans will likely expand well beyond the established markets of the Sentara providers, which will weaken the vertical linkages that exist between Sentara (the base provider) and its health plans.

Kaiser Health Plan and a number of other group and staff model HMOs have achieved high levels of geographic compatibility between vertically integrated plan and provider partners. This is largely because Kaiser is an HMO company first and a provider company second. As a result, Kaiser invests only in the provider capacity it needs to support its changing beneficiary numbers. In California, for example, Kaiser has been able to plan its hospital investments carefully in every case, reflecting growing or declining penetration of its HMO business. In markets where Kaiser has much less penetration and where significant local resistance exists against Kaiser building its own hospitals (especially outside of its California and Hawaii markets), Kaiser has simply dropped the hospital portion from its vertical arrangements.

A lack of strategic fit between HMO and provider businesses, however, was clear in the case of Humana Inc. As discussed in Strategy Note 9.1, having evolved into a vertical model in the 1980s, Humana immediately encountered the complications of integrating its two businesses for which the markets were not at all compatible with one another. The following anecdote summarizes the kinds of strategic fit problems that Humana encountered when it tried to establish its HMO business within the same communities where it had its own hospitals.

STRATEGY NOTE 9.1. HUMANA: COMPLICATIONS WITH VERTICAL

Source: Data from Conrad, D. A., and G. A. Hoare. 1994. *Strategic Alignment: Manging Integrated Health Systems*. Chicago: Health Administration Press, and from Humana's web site: http://www.humana.com/corporatecomm/companyinfo/history.asp.

From being one of the first and largest vertically integrated healthcare systems, Humana is now only in the health insurance business. In the 1970s and early 1980s, Humana was a functionally and regionally structured hospital company, offering many services, including administration, billing, and information technology, centralized at corporate headquarters in Louisville, Kentucky.

As Humana added physician and managed care services, the company became a divisionally organized company (see Chapter 10 for a discussion of organization structure and strategy). In 1993, Humana divested its 75 hospitals (forming a company by the name of Galen, which then became the first major acquisition consummated by Columbia in 1994; see this discussion in Chapter 8) and became a national managed care company. Humana faced a number of problems that motivated the company to divest its hospital business, most of which involved conflicting economic objectives between managed care, hospital, and physician businesses that are inherent in vertical arrangements.

One major problem involved conflicts between the health insurance and provider businesses (see the discussion later in this chapter on lack of strategic fit). The purpose of a health insurance company is to sell insurance policies by keeping its premium prices low. The best way to control expenses is to minimize customers' use of healthcare services, mostly by lowering the incidence and length of hospitalization. In contrast, healthcare providers increase their economic wealth by increasing utilization.

A second problem had to do with transfer pricing. The insurance plan had an incentive to contract with non-Humana hospitals, if they offered lower prices. However, like many vertically integrated companies, Humana used transfer prices to compute the sale of its hospital services to its insurance division. Generally, transfer pricing may be set at full charges, cost of goods, or at some discounted rate. But Humana set the transfer prices for its own hospitals higher than the market prices for other competitive hospitals. As a result, Humana's insurance division often preferred to refer its patients to non-Humana hospitals.

A third problem was Humana's troubled relationships with its physicians. Predominantly, Humana relied on an individual practice association (IPA) model, which is an HMO model that contracts with a network of doctors through its IPAs. However, because the doctors were in private practices, they did not necessarily operate in Humana's best interests (a problem common to most nongroup or staff-model HMOs). Like other HMOs in the industry, Humana tried to trim costs by cutting the amount of money it paid its doctors, which caused many of the doctors to retaliate by referring patients to competitor hospitals. Humana's two businesses (managed care and hospital) thus worked at extreme cross-purposes.

Another physician problem surfaced with those doctors who were not selected to be on Humana's HMO panels. Having been excluded from the panels, these physicians tended to retaliate by referring patients to non-Humana hospitals. In response, Humana began to welcome these physicians, but this created yet another problem: Humana had diminished its power to influence physician behavior. After all, Humana's health insurance plan was not a significant factor for many of these doctors because the plan covered only a few of their patients. Humana thus had little leverage over those doctors. This lack of incentive and influence led to physician indifference and a tendency to increase the number of hospital days used by Humana enrollees (a problem for the HMO). Worse, many of those days were spent in non-Humana facilities.

A fourth problem is that Humana hospital costs grew primarily because the hospital division's management lacked experience in the new businesses. David Jones started the health insurance division precisely because of a need to fill many empty Humana hospital beds. The salaried physicians in their owned primary care centers did little to enhance referrals to Humana hospitals. Humana's tightly centralized hospital management had no experience in guiding salaried physician practices and

could offer little advice to their physician managers. Perhaps because the physicians earned the same salary regardless of the actual number of patients they saw, many of them failed to develop
a patient following in their communities. As an owner rather
than a renter, Humana was also forced to pay the full costs of
the hospitals and its salaried physicians whether they were used
or not. As a renter, in contrast, Humana would have had the lux-
ury of paying for hospitals only when it needed them and at bar-
gain rates to boot.

In the early 1990s, Humana found that owning both HMOs
and hospitals put it at a disadvantage when contract signing time
came. Jones said, "After the strategies began to appear to some
extent incompatible, we starting having trouble carrying water
on both shoulders. It seemed that if we solved a problem for the
hospital it would create a problem with the health plan, and
[vice versa]. We could see that conflict, but amazingly enough,
it did not surface for a number of years. We started in 1983 being
an integrated company, and the strategy worked reasonably well
for a while. But it got more difficult as we got larger, which surprised me. I would have thought it would have gotten easier as
we got larger."

Humana used to be one of the most powerful players in the
healthcare industry. But a series of ill-advised managerial decisions, including the company's attempt to move into a vertical
model and its inability to shift gears as quickly as managed care
was accelerating, all spelled doom for the one-time hospital and
insurance king. Even after the divestiture of its hospital business, Humana took years to realign its profitability. Humana hit
rock bottom in the second quarter of 1996 when it suffered a
net loss of $95 million after taking a $200 million pre-tax charge
to keep its new Washington, DC, operation in business. In 1999,
losses resulted in large part from a previously announced fourth-
quarter charge of $495 million relating to the write-off of good-
will and the sale of devalued assets.

Humana has been working to revitalize its flagging financials.
Since suffering a $382 million loss in 1999, the company has cut
administrative expenses, boosted premiums, and divested non-
core operations. It has dropped its workers' compensation unit,
two money-losing HMOs, and part of its Medicaid business.

When it entered Richmond, Virginia, in the mid-1980s, Humana came face to face with the strategic fit problem. To kick off its new product, Humana convened a meeting at a local hotel, to which the business community of Richmond was invited. First, Humana made the claim that it could beat the price of the dominant, local managed care provider by as much as 20 percent, which created a hopeful buzz among prospective clients in the audience. During the question-and-answer session, however, the weaknesses in the plan became evident. At that time, Humana had only one hospital in Richmond—St. Luke's—which was located on the northwest side of town. The vertical model called for the beneficiaries, regardless of where they lived, to use that one hospital.

Right away, the employer representatives began asking how employees located on the south side of the James River could possibly get to St. Luke's on the north side. Questions were also raised about the employees' physicians, most of whom were unlikely to have admitting privileges at St. Luke's. With these questions, the glaring flaws in Humana's vertical design were exposed. In general, the geographic reach of Humana's health plan far exceeded that of its hospital, thus negating any real benefit attributable to a vertical arrangement.

One other prominent example of the strategic fit problem is the 1994 vertical merger between two major Minneapolis players, which formed Allina. At that time, the leading local hospital organization, HealthSpan (which is itself the product of several mergers between other local multihospital systems), merged with Medica, a successful HMO operating out of Minneapolis. At the time, this merger was viewed as a vertical model for the country. As time passed, however, flaws in Allina's vertical structure became more and more visible. Significantly, the market positions of the two organizations were not well fitted nor were their respective incentives. By the end of the 1990s, Medica admitted less than a third of its patients to the Allina hospitals. Medica even had to pay premiums to some of Allina's physicians to induce them to admit to the Allina hospitals. In the end, the hospital revenues coming from Medica were less than 20 percent of its totals.

The lack of strategic fit, conflicting objectives, and failure to integrate management across the major components of Allina all led to the ultimate demise and disbanding of the merger in 2001. This case is an especially important example because it illustrates the extreme difficulty encountered when provider systems attempt to forward integrate locally into the managed care business. The Humana example illustrates the same issues for the merger between two nationally expanded companies.

Competing with Customers

A second major problem or limitation with vertical integration is that it can bring providers into direct competition with their clients, and health-care is particularly susceptible to this problem because of its structures of payment and delivery. Hospitals that forward integrate will be competing with the very managed care companies with which they have contracts. In response, those companies can be expected to retaliate by shifting their contracts to rival providers or not agreeing to favorable deals with the integrating hospital organizations.

When it entered the managed care business in 1984, Sentara faced little retaliation from managed care companies. Not only was the managed care market poorly organized in Norfolk at the time but also Sentara already enjoyed a fairly dominant position in its market, making it difficult for any managed care company to countervail Sentara's move into the managed care business. The situation was quite different for another Virginia company located just a few hundred miles to the north of Norfolk—INOVA Health System. In the 1980s, INOVA also had aspirations of entering the managed care market; its situation, however, differed significantly from that of Sentara. Located in the northern Virginia side of the Washington, DC, metropolitan area, INOVA enjoyed a strong position in the hospital market. Only one other major player—HCA—competed with its hospitals on the Virginia side of DC. At the time, HCA had three hospitals and INOVA had three. Significantly, however, Kaiser Health Plan had become well established in the area; in fact, it had a major contract with INOVA. Obviously, the prospect that INOVA might compete with them was not well received by Kaiser. Anecdotal evidence suggests that Kaiser threatened to shift some of its business to HCA if INOVA moved into managed care, which for this and other reasons, INOVA did not.

Hospitals' gains in market power over the past decade might tempt them to reconsider vertical integration once again. In any case, growing evidence indicates that the strong local systems are fully willing to use their new-found market clout to negotiate with managed care companies (Strunk, Devers, and Hurley 2001). In time, these systems can test their powers still further by moving downstream into managed care, even if this means that they would come into direct competition with some of their most important managed care clients.

Confounded Strategic Alignments

The final strategic limitation of vertical integration pertains to the integration of hospital and physician businesses (Conrad and Dowling 1990), a strategy that many hospitals and hospital systems attempted in the 1990s and with which they encountered serious management and strategic problems (Walston, Kimberly, and Burns 1996). On the other hand, the American Hospital Association (2000) data indicate that by 1999 nearly 45 percent of hospitals mentioned that they or their health systems were directly involved in one or more of a variety of physician arrangements, ranging from foundation models to IPAs. However, this finding is likely to be a significant overstatement of the degree to which hospitals are seriously involved in true vertical arrangements with physicians.

Note that virtually all attempts by hospitals to integrate with physicians have taken place at the local level, between one or more local hospitals and selected members of their medical staffs. Thus, a central challenge presented by such arrangements is a confounding of the relationships between local hospitals and their physicians (Luke and Walston 2003). The physicians usually retain significant professional power, even after their practices have been acquired. This factor often seriously weakens a hospital or hospital system's ability to control owned physicians and ultimately to carry out its strategic objectives. The diversity of ways in which hospitals and physicians are interrelated distinguishes this particular combination from most other multibusiness combinations in other industries. This diversity can be of such consequence that, if not carefully evaluated, it can seriously compromise a system's vertical or other strategic agenda. Luke and Walston (2003) identified at least six distinctive market relationships that exist between physicians and hospitals.

1. *Physicians and hospitals are often direct competitors of each other.* This occurs especially in the competitive struggle over the provision of ancillary services, which is often confounded by the fact that certain physicians are members of hospitals' voluntary medical staffs. Thus, hospitals that confront their physicians in the marketplace through vertical integration with other physicians or through other business ventures risk undermining the delicate balance they have with their referring and admitting physicians. Hospitals, which are usually better capitalized and managed than are physician organizations, usually take the initiative in developing new services, whether offered internally or externally. In pursuing such ventures, hospitals easily run afoul of their medical staffs, who themselves might be considering business ventures in these areas. Such conflicts can also easily undermine any budding vertical arrangements that hospitals might be contemplating.

2. *Physicians and hospitals function as substitutes for one another.* Care offered by hospitals (e.g., with nurse anesthetists) can displace the care that might be offered by independent specialists (e.g., anesthesiologists).

3. *Physicians and hospitals are often joint producers of services.* Physicians, who otherwise are independent practitioners, serve within hospitals by directing the patient care delivered there. Typically, a similar arrangement in nearly any other industry would not be possible, as the independent professional would be immediately given employee status.

4. *Physicians and hospitals function as complements to one another* (see Brandenburger and Nalebuff 1996 for the concept of complements). This occurs, for example, when hospitals and physicians join up to negotiate global contracts with managed care plans.

5. *Physicians and hospitals share the same regulatory environment.* Therefore, they share responsibilities for quality, risk management, and error control. Also, they can share threats from malpractice.

6. *Physicians and hospitals relate to one another vertically.* Even this type of relationship is confounded because it is not easy to determine which of the two is the buyer and which is the seller. In fact, they each play both roles. Luke and Walston characterized this as *bidirectional vertical*, reflecting the bidirectional flows that occur between physicians and hospitals. The relationships are not precisely vertical because only limited financial exchange occurs between the two parties. Insurance companies function as the third party, handling payment. On the other hand, patients and services do flow between them. Primary care physicians, in effect functioning as suppliers, send referrals to hospitals and to hospital-based physicians. Hospitals buy or acquire the services of physicians to treat the hospital's patients. Physicians also buy or send their patients to hospitals to obtain ancillary services.

Overall, the physician-hospital relationships are muddled, highly complex, and very delicate. Certainly, viewing the interplay between hospitals and physicians as strictly vertical is unreasonable. From a transaction cost economics perspective, however, the degree of complexity and challenge inherent in their exchange relationships suggests that some form of integration would make a great deal of sense. Even with all of the foregoing complications, however, the problem of strategic fit exists. Physicians do not have complete control over which hospital is selected for the care of their patients. For this reason, they often maintain multiple staff privileges across hospitals, many of which are competitors to one another.

Finally, there is the problem that the "informal" network that binds primary and specialist physicians together may not align well with the network established within a formal, hospital-initiated vertical arrangement. So long as the physician sector remains fragmented, referral structures are likely to remain informal, in which case aligning the strategic interests of physicians and hospitals can be a formidable task. On the other hand, the managed care companies have been formalizing and shifting around the referral arrangements by selectively including physicians in their health plan panels. Thus, the complications associated with interfering with informal referral and colleague networks might by now have been greatly diminished.

If the physician markets were to become more concentrated, however, the structure of interrelationships could shift in ways that diminish or enhance the complexities inherent in physician-hospital integration. But how? The Los Angeles and Minneapolis markets provide some hint on what can result from physicians forming into organized groups and then combining with hospital systems. The relative market power of many large physician groups in Los Angeles match up fairly well with the market power of local hospital players. As a result of their market strength, the physician groups have competed directly with the hospital systems for control of managed care contracts. In a few cases, they have even acquired their own hospitals. Although the acquisition has not resulted in much vertical integration between physician and hospital organizations, it does offer a different prospect for integration between them. Large physician groups, in other words, potentially can internalize many of the structural complexities presented in cases where hospitals align with individual physicians and small physician group practices. Thus, combinations between large hospital systems and large physician groups might be like the typical vertical arrangement seen in other industries.

Physician groups are also very strong in the Minneapolis market, but so too are the hospital and the managed care systems in that area. The strategic maneuvering of powerful players there has, by contrast to Los Angeles, produced mostly vertical arrangements between physician, hospital, and managed care companies. One of Allina's major competitors in Minneapolis is HealthPartners, a staff and group model vertically integrated system. In earlier years, both HealthPartners and Allina joined physicians, hospitals, and health plans. The two systems differed, however, in that the former was essentially a physician-based system and the latter a hospital-initiated system. HealthPartners is therefore more like Kaiser in the sense that the hospital component does not control the system's agenda.

The key point here is that both of the Minneapolis vertical integration examples represent the possibility of combining large physician and hospital organizations. As physician organizations get larger, the industry might find more ways to accomplish what many think is the inevitable vertical restructuring that is needed in healthcare.

CONCLUSION

This chapter addresses possibly the most interesting strategy in healthcare—vertical integration. It is interesting because it seems a rational approach for delivering costly health services, but at the same time it presents significant limitations when applied to this highly institutionalized industry. Vertical integration can be the most complex and costly of all strategies: it carries a complex array of advantages, drawbacks, and risks that can easily affect the survivability of any organizations that attempt it. Thus, a strategy analyst must fully understand all of the factors surrounding this strategy before engaging in it. These factors include the circumstances in the market; the capabilities and prospects of the potential organizations to be integrated; the likely responses from rivals, including buyers and sellers; and the administrative infrastructure required in facilitating the internalized transactions of the strategy. Seeds of failure can be found in any one of these factors.

Still, some healthcare organizations have successfully implemented vertical integration. Vertical works best in markets in which the prospective partners are large or dominant. Because they already enjoy strong market positions and established organizational structures, such systems are better able to mollify buyer reactions, navigate physician-hospital relationships, and manage complex interrelationships inherent in this strategy. They are also more likely to be able to draw on their established market and organizational strengths, which help them weather the uncertainties of transitioning to a vertical model. Regional models (discussed in Chapter 8) might also be well positioned to align the market demands of HMOs, which need room for growth, with the sprawling geographic distributions of their coordinated and possibly integrated provider networks.

Despite its diverse challenges, many healthcare organizations will surely be tempted to try vertical in the years to come. Those that discover the keys to unlocking its potential can gain significant early-mover advantages. Unfortunately, the other obvious possibility is that those keys will not be found, and the many risks associated with vertical integration will overwhelm those who attempt it.

REFERENCES

American Hospital Association. 2000. *1999 American Hospital Association Annual Survey of Hospitals*. Chicago: Health Forum/AHA.

Aventis. 2001. *Managed Care Digest* Series. [Online information; retrieved 1/03.] http://www.managedcaredigest.com/.

Brandenburger, A. M., and B. J. Nalebuff. 1996. *Co-opetition*. New York: Doubleday.

Conrad, D. A., and W. Dowling. 1990. "Vertical Integration in Health Services: Theory and Managerial Implications." *Health Care Management Review* 15 (Fall): 9–33.

Conrad, D. A., and G. A. Hoare. 1994. *Strategic Alignment: Managing Integrated Health Systems*. Chicago: Health Administration Press.

Conrad, D. A., and S. M. Shortell. 1996. "Integrated Health Services: Promises and Performance." *Frontiers of Health Services Management* 13 (1): 3–40.

Enthoven, A. C. 1980. *Health Plan: The Only Practical Solution to the Soaring Cost of Medical Care*. Boston: Addison-Wesley.

Harrigan, K. R. 1983. *Strategies for Vertical Integration*. Lexington, MA: Lexington Books.

Jones, A. 1987. *The Art of War in the Western World*. New York: Oxford University Press.

Luke, R. D., and S. Walston. 2003. "Strategy in an Institutional Environment: Lessons Learned from the 90s 'Revolution' in Health Care." In *Advances in Health Care Organization Theory*, edited by S. S. Mick, M. Wyttenbach, and associates. San Francisco: Jossey-Bass.

Mick, S. 1990. "Explaining Vertical Integration in Health Care: An Analysis and Synthesis of Transaction-Cost Economics and Strategic Management Theory." In *Innovations in Health Care Delivery: Insights for Organization Theory*, edited by S. Mick, 207–40. San Francisco: Jossey-Bass.

Mick, S. S., and D. A. Conrad. 1988. "The Decision to Integrate Vertically in Health Care Organizations." *Hospital & Health Services Administration* 33 (3): 345–60.

Ouchi, W. G. 1977. "Review of Markets and Hierarchies." *Administrative Science Quarterly* 22: 541–44.

Porter, M. E. 1980. *Competitive Strategy*. New York: The Free Press.

————. 1985. *Competitive Advantage: Creating and Sustaining Superior Performance*. New York: The Free Press.

Strunk, B. C., K. Devers, and R. H. Hurley. 2001. *Health Plan–Provider Showdowns on the Rise*, Issue Brief no. 40. Washington, DC: Center for Studying Health System Change.

Walston, S. L., J. R. Kimberly, and L. R. Burns. 1996. "Owned Vertical Integration and Health Care Promise and Performance." *Health Care Management Review* 21 (Winter): 83–92.

Williamson, O. E. 1975. *Markets and Hierarchies, Analysis and Antitrust Implications: A Study in the Economics of Internal Organization*. New York: The Free Press.

————. 1986. *Economic Organization: Firms, Markets and Policy Controls*. New York: New York University Press.

Chapter 10

Organizational Structure

The staff needs of a commander of a concentrated army of 40,000 men differed markedly from those of 200,000 spread over a wide area. The Prussian army developed a larger staff composed of men who had received uniform training, so that all had the same doctrine and vocabulary. Serving on the staffs of army and corps commanders, these officers understood one another readily and gave their commanders consistent recommendations, coordinated by a chief who could represent their views to the commander, the staff could provide counsel and carry out the commander's orders .... Coordination and management improved because of harmony and communication between the staffs at different command levels....
—*Jones (1987, 392)*

As organizations compete in today's changing environment, their ability to align structures, business strategies, and management practices with conditions in their markets becomes critical for sustaining and enhancing competitive advantage (Porter 1985). Failure to achieve such alignment can cause organizations to

- lose sales and market share,
- incur increasing costs and inefficiencies,
- generate discontent among customers and suppliers,
- engender internal organizational conflict, and
- lose strategic direction.

Effective management requires both the positioning of the organization in the external environment (power and position strategies) and the internal systems and resources (potential and performance strategies). It also requires choices to be made regarding the timing of strategic moves and the degree of risk an organization is willing to assume, both of which relate to pace strategies. The structure adopted by an organization can have a major impact on all such organizational choices.

Many factors are involved in organizational design, including the structure or the arrangement and placement of functional duties within an organization, the flow of information, and the level and locus of decision making. These and other factors contribute to the efficiency, effectiveness, and quality of organizational decision making and the accomplishment of strategic objectives. In this chapter, we discuss the relationship between organizational structure and strategy. Specifically, we examine four major structural forms: functional, divisional, matrix, and virtual. Our purpose for this chapter is to examine structure in a strategic context, not to provide a comprehensive coverage of issues relating to organizational structure.

In terms of the five Ps of competitive advantage, the structuring of organizations falls somewhere between potential and performance. To the extent that structure establishes unique capabilities, it falls in the category of potential. To the extent that it facilitates greater organizational control and improvements in efficiency, it can be better classified as performance. Regardless of its role, organizational structure should be viewed as more than a matter of organizational design. For most complex organizations, organizational structure often determines how completely they are able to achieve competitive advantage. As noted later in the chapter, the fact that many healthcare organizations have adopted loose organizational forms to accomplish high strategic purposes can be construed as either a significant flaw or an advantage, depending on one's perspective. It can be considered a flaw if the loose structures did not facilitate sufficient control and coordination. It is an advantage, however, if it enabled organizations to move into strategic alignments earlier (and to exit them earlier as well) than is possible with considerably tighter structures.

ORGANIZATIONAL STRUCTURE BASICS

Organizational structure has been a major consideration at the level of practice. In fact, many organizations expend vast resources annually on reorganizing and restructuring. Some seem to cycle through different structures, changing frequently from one structural form to another. Unfortunately, as Rumelt (1974, 149) said, "structure...follows fashion," a point that is especially germane to healthcare because of the key role institutional influences play in determining organizational strategies and structural form. The healthcare strategy analyst thus must take special care to understand the interrelationships between organizational structure and the accomplishment of strategic objectives or risk being led by fashion more than function.

Modern organizational structure developed concurrently with the Industrial Revolution. Many early structures were developed to coordinate large military ventures and, later, to facilitate the new productivity demands of the Industrial Revolution. In the 1700s, the era of Adam Smith (British philosopher and economist), individuals were trained in all aspects of production processes. Craftsmen would not only produce their products but also handle purchasing, marketing, and selling functions. Adam Smith found that productivity increased substantially by breaking labor into components and distributing tasks more widely among workers. Complex and formal structures thus evolved as organizations became too large for individuals to manage the increasing number and complexities of tasks. All of the new structural forms facilitated divisions of labor and organizational control, both of which were needed for the management of growing organizational complexity. Under the new organizational forms, specific duties tended to be prescribed. For example, in pin making, one drew out wire, another straightened it, a third cut it, a fourth pointed it, and a fifth grinded it into a head. According to Smith (1910, 5), "But if they had all wrought separately and independently, and without any of them having been educated to this peculiar business, they certainly could not each have made 20, perhaps not one pin, in a day."

Such divisions of labor have had profound effects on the functioning of many organizations. How labor is organized and tasks and decisions are divided up and coordinated can affect all aspects of an organization. It can influence the quality of organizational decisions, impede or facilitate the flow of information, and affect the attainment of economies of scale. In addition, it can affect the degree to which an organization's strategies are achieved. See Strategy Note 10.1 for a clear example of how structure, management skill, and strategy were integrally interrelated in a major healthcare system.

STRUCTURAL FORMS

Most organizations use one of three *structural forms* (or some combination of these): functional, multidivisional, and matrix organizations. In this section, these structural forms, as well as their relationships to market strategy, are discussed. A novel organizational approach that is adopted by a number of forming healthcare systems—the virtual organization—is also examined.

Functional Organizations

Functional organizations are structured by common tasks, services, or roles. Hospitals have traditionally adopted functional structures, which have even extended to the executive office by the designation of vice presidents (or

STRATEGY NOTE 10.1. THE CASE OF CENTURA HEALTH SYSTEM: A FAILURE TO ALIGN STRUCTURE AND STRATEGY

In 1995, Centura Health System underwent a major change in strategy. It radically restructured and centralized much decision-making power within its corporate office in Denver, Colorado. However, after only three years, the organization was forced to revise its strategy. It quickly decentralized many functional services that had been centralized only a few years before.

Centura was formed in 1995 in response to an expected growth in capitation payment (which most predicted would represent 70 percent of payment in their markets but at its height never got higher than 30 percent) and in the increasing power of Columbia/HCA (which was a correct assumption as the organization, now called HCA, currently has around 40 percent market share in Denver, compared to Centura's 20 percent). Believing that it "had to skate where the puck" was, Centura formed integrated delivery systems within its major markets that was composed of its own HMO, owned physician networks, and its hospital system. Centura also jumped into direct contracting and took full risk. Most of these ventures experienced financial difficulties.

To accomplish their objectives, Centura's leaders felt that most service functions (recruiting, finance, dietary, and so on) needed to be centralized. It did not take long, however, for observers to conclude that the centralized corporate personnel were too removed from the hospitals and had lost sight of their core business—patient care. Because of losses in the HMO and physician businesses, Centura pushed all of the hospitals to reduce costs. In one year, the leadership asked for a 20 percent cost reduction, which included a cutback of hospital management teams as well. At one of Centura's largest hospitals, from 1995 to 1997, the number of directors shrank from 90 to 21 and the number of vice presidents from 12 to 2.

The leadership felt that the only way to beat Columbia/HCA was to be more like that organization, which meant copying Columbia/HCA's structure and centralizing many decisions.

Centura's leaders began making many decisions with limited input from the hospital level regarding HMO contracting, purchasing physician practices, and structuring hospital services. The result was not as they had hoped. Contracting and services became fairly Denver-centric and provided only limited help to Centura's out-of-Denver hospitals.

Communications between the hospitals and corporate were weak. The leadership did not visit the hospitals perhaps as much as they should have in those years. The local hospital administrators had limited authority to communicate corporate information to local hospitals' board members, a situation that contributed to a degree of estrangement among those members. Recruiting was likewise centralized at the corporate level, even though the roles and personnel at corporate changed frequently. Hospital and corporate personnel had a compensation system that encouraged further centralization. Bonuses, for example, were provided based on annual performance. Hospital personnel felt that they were forced to support corporate decisions or face possible termination. People became less willing to ask difficult questions.

Instead of saving money, overhead allocations to the hospitals dramatically increased. Allocations to the largest hospital, for example, more than doubled to $27 million from $13 million. At the same time, the annual amount of capital to purchase equipment given to this hospital declined to $4 million from $18 million. During this difficult financial period, the corporation hired a plethora of consultants to resolve the losses, including Aslax, Ernst & Young, APM, Andersen, and the Hunter Group. Hospital personnel later commented that they could not think of one thing that the string of consultants introduced except for more work. As a result of the consultants' demands and the poor access to data (all data had to be obtained from the corporate office and little were available), the middle managers went into survivor mode. They prepared and kept their own databases, which could be reformatted when required by the next batch of new consultants. Silos that were thought to be broken sprang up anew, as individuals and groups tried to protect their remaining turf.

Centralized decisions also affected employee morale. One of the large hospitals had an established gain-sharing program and, as a result of positive improvement, had accrued $500,000 in 1995 for employee bonuses. However, after this was announced to the hospital employees, corporate intervened, stating that because all of their hospitals did not have this benefit, none should. The system then went to flat, across-the-board increases or none at all. At the same time, other competitors were giving bonuses to their employees; as a result, a number of the system's best employees left to work for the competitors. Corporate also wanted to systematize the identification of all of their hospitals. All were required to remove their local identities and to brand the hospitals with the Centura name. Hospital signs and identifications that many had used for more than 100 years were taken down. Employees were told to answer phones with a greeting from Centura, which tended to confuse patients, physicians, and employees.

The bottom line is that Centura's corporate leadership was restructured in 1998, and most of the services were decentralized back to the hospital level. The Hunter Group was then brought in for about one year, and its recommended changes seemed to work magic. In 1999, the largest hospital in the system lost $4.5 million (after a huge corporate overhead allocation) and the corporation lost $60 million. Two years later (June 2001), that same hospital made $30 million and the corporation made $141 million.

What a difference a year, and some much needed corporate restructuring, can make!

some equivalent title) for marketing, finance, nursing, and other departments. Functional divisions also occur at various depths and breadths within organizations, including within departments, strategic business units, and corporate headquarters.

The advantage of a functional design remains the same as was described long ago by Adam Smith: the specialization of expertise and the potential for capturing economies of scale. A healthcare system, for example, might centralize managed care, marketing, finance, support services, and nursing in separate organizational divisions. The managed care division can be more effective at negotiating contracts for the whole system rather than delegating responsibility for such negotiations to each individual facility. Marketing might obtain better price concessions on placement of advertising as well as achieve lower production costs by centralizing functions and negotiating over the volumes of work. Finance might be able to afford more sophisticated information technologies and thereby generate more cost-effective billings. Functional centralization might also facilitate more focused control over the formulation and implementation of market strategies. One widely recognized example of a company that gains considerable competitive advantage from functional structuring is Wal-Mart, Inc. Wal-Mart locates its stores in many areas, including smaller towns and suburbs. It uses the specialized talents of planners, logistics specialists, and store personnel to support this network of stores and to create one of the most efficient inventory and distribution systems in the country.

Centralization using a functional form, however, can produce some negative effects. It can, for example, lead to the formation of silos, which introduce conflicting goals across functional areas, encourage the growth of subcultures, and put up artificial information barriers. Individual functional units in organizations often become more interested in achieving their own particular goals than those of the organization as a whole. Often, such units form their own values, vocabularies, and behavioral norms, a situation that further reinforces the separation between units and creates tension and mistrust within the organization. These types of differences often preclude communication of information and delay timely or effective implementation of decisions. Functionally specialized individuals might believe (sometimes with justification) that information they possess will not be understood by members located in other functional areas, thus encouraging them to withhold data, believing that the data might otherwise lead to misunderstandings, inefficiencies, and lost productivity.

All of these factors can be critically important in strategic decision making given that many strategies require considerable and often highly coordinated organizational effort for successful implementation. This is even truer in highly volatile and competitive markets, where a lack of coordination can spell disaster as the environment might shift faster than can the strategies of a structurally constrained organization. In fact, information overload attributable to organizational growth and the increasing demand for product variety and market responsiveness is a major reason that many organizations abandon the functional model (Chandler 1962).

In relatively small organizations, including freestanding hospitals and most physician group practices, decision making and information might appropriately be centralized functionally, typically within executive offices. Detailed decisions involving product improvement, product design, capital allocation, personnel, and even mergers and acquisitions can be made quickly under a centralized, functional structure. However, the effectiveness of functional centralization generally declines as organizations grow. Exponentially increasing numbers of decisions and quantities of information, which often accompany organizational growth, easily overwhelm functional areas. For this reason, many large corporations in the 1940s and 1950s (e.g., General Motors) reorganized into multidivisional organizational structures (Miles and Snow 1992).

Functional organization limitations formed the basis for Mintzberg's critique of strategic planning. He noted that the typical strategic planning structure divided decision making between "performance control" functions (objectives setting and budget planning) and "action planning" functions (strategic decision making and program planning). The expectation within strategic planning is that considerable information flow and coordination occurs horizontally across functional areas. Unfortunately, as he effectively argued, such functions have tended to become isolated from one another (the silo effect) and, as a result, have failed to achieve the coordination in decision making envisaged in the formularized strategic planning models. Mintzberg (1994, 78–81) characterized this separation between the primary action and performance functions as "the great divide of planning."

Multidivisional Organizations

Multidivisional organizations congregate multiple functional tasks within miniorganizations, which then operate relatively autonomously. In the past, divisional structures were seen to be superior to functional form in managing the information-overload problem that often occurs with growth (Chandler 1962). Typically, multidivisional organizations decentralize decision making to the business units, thereby allowing the corporate office to concentrate its focus on corporate strategy, capital allocation, and monitoring of the operational and strategic performance of business units (see Chapter 6). This creates the advantage of increasing accountability, given that common/comparable measures can be established across different divisions and internal competition for available capital can be stimulated. The ability to allocate and allow competition for internal capital is believed by some to be a main advantage of a multidivisional organization. For example, Williamson (1975, 147–48) stated

[Cash flows] are not automatically returned to their sources but instead are exposed to an internal competition. Investment proposals from the several divisions are solicited and evaluated by the general management...this assignment of cash flows to high yield uses is the most fundamental attribute of the [multidivisional] enterprise.

Because of this advantage, the multidivisional structure has been widely used to manage portfolio- and conglomerate-model organizations. In general, however, this structure fits well any organization that diversifies into multibusiness or multimarket activities (see Chapter 8), especially if little coordination is required between the businesses or between markets. On the other hand, if interdivision coordination is important, then the multidivisional structure alone might not be ideal.

Clearly, the multidivisional structure has disadvantages. First, there is the problem of duplication of services—that is, redundant marketing, manufacturing, and other functional services that are established within each unit. Costs can escalate when functions are repeated in multiple areas. Likewise, the quality of functions performed within divisions can vary widely and the level of expertise can be diluted. Second, decentralized divisions easily become isolated, and competition for capital allocation can readily deteriorate into destructive interdivisional conflicts, in which information is withheld and resources are not shared across divisions. Division-specific incentives, such as compensation or promotion, can accentuate this negative competition. Managers may even try to one-up their peers and maintain a resource-scarce mentality that can lead to poor corporatewide results. All of the foregoing can damage competitive advantage if not prevented.

Although multidivisional structures encourage local adaptation to market forces, they also diminish the standardization of processes and products and the seamlessness of the corporation. For example, many of the retail companies that created separate Internet divisions to facilitate adaptation to the rapidly changing web-based markets ran into conflicts with their established businesses. For example, in 2000, Sears created an Internet store that carried a somewhat different inventory than did the physical stores. Thus, customers calling the Internet store about Sears store products were often told to call the local stores. Also, many products purchased on the

Internet could not be returned to local Sears stores. This divisional separation therefore might have facilitated better market adaptation, but the lack of unity created by this arrangement produced poor customer service and considerable confusion in the marketplace.

Corporate executives in decentralized organizations can too easily distance themselves from their divisional operations and thus find that they lack the needed insights and skills to understand their disparate businesses. Corporate leaders can also focus so much on capital allocation and corporate strategy (e.g., mergers, divestitures, acquisitions) that they lose touch with the operational side of their businesses. Adding to this difficulty, the leaders might find that they rarely visit their divisions and therefore lose sight of their core services. Without vigilance, corporate executives can easily find themselves lacking key insights and knowledge that might cripple their strategic decision making.

Many examples of these kinds of problems can be found at a local level in the hospital sector. Reengineering efforts, for example, have led some hospitals to decentralize services, such as phlebotomy and respiratory therapy, to the departmental level, treating the departments as lower-level business units. When such services are spread among different nursing units, cross-coverage and maintenance of skill levels often become problems because there is often insufficient demand at the departmental level to support high levels of specialization. This can lead to other problems as well, including increased competition and conflict between departments; a lack of standardization and consistency across departments; and a greater distance of top executives from operations, which results in poor managerial expertise and day-to-day oversight.

Transfer pricing can also create negative organizational effects. When businesses have separate divisions and transfer materials or services between units, a method for accounting for the cost of this exchange must be developed. Three general methods for transfer pricing are available, all of which potentially have negative side effects: (1) payment of full market prices, (2) payment of market prices less a discount, and (3) payment of costs—marginal or some type of full cost. The method that is selected for transfer prices can have deleterious effects by discouraging intracompany exchange.

Transfer pricing, for example, contributed to an interdivisional problem encountered by Humana, which in the 1990s was a vertically integrated hospital and managed care company (see Strategy Note 9.1 in Chapter 9).

The Divisions Within Multidivisional Structures

Multidivisional organizations are usually divided in one of two ways:

1. Products
2. Geography

Dividing by product (called a *product-line division*) has been common in many multiproduct organizations, such as Sears, General Mills, and DuPont. Healthcare product-line divisions might focus on cardiology, oncology, women's service, or pediatrics, or more broadly on acute care, long-term care, or managed care. *Geographic division* in healthcare reflects the movement by many provider organizations into multiple markets. The basis that healthcare organizations use to create divisions depends on a number of factors:

- the organization's overall scale and scope,
- the organization's geographic configuration, and
- other distinctive organizational and market characteristics.

Dividing an organization by products can produce economies of scale and increase quality and reputation. For example, a number of healthcare organizations have initiated ventures to create heart hospitals, which concentrate cardiac services within separate hospitals. The extensive capital required to construct these facilities has been justified by a significant reduction in patient length of stay and by improved quality attributable to higher concentrations of professionals and skills that focus solely on cardiac care. An interesting way to conceptualize product-line divisions in some hospitals is to designate divisions as hospitals within a hospital, thereby connoting a stand-alone characteristic for each such division. In the 1990s, applications of two very popular managerial innovations—reengineering and patient-centered care—contributed to a trend in redistributing into subunits a number of functional tasks that were traditionally centralized in hospitals (Hammer and Champy 1993; Lathrop 1993). Patient services such as phlebotomy, respiratory therapy, and housekeeping were organized around nursing units. Sometimes, only the reporting relationships changed, while separate specialized positions were retained. In other cases, the traditional duties were segmented into new positions, such as clinical associates, that combined many of these functions (Walston and Kimberly 1997).

In general, dividing by geography makes sense when distinct competitive, political, legal, cultural, and other differences exist across markets. (On a very broad scale, multinational divisions of global companies are often organized by geography for just such reasons.) Prior to the 1990s, information barriers were significant factors in driving large organizations to adopt multidivisional, geographically based structures. However, with the advent of high-speed data transmission, these barriers have become somewhat less significant in determining organizational design, although large distances among units still sustain high information barriers. On the other hand, if an organization were much less geographically dispersed, the frequency of interaction among supervisory personnel and the quality and amount of key information exchanged might increase. This interrelationship between geographic proximity and divisional structuring is a major strategic concern within the provider sector of healthcare, primarily because of the great potential for integration that close proximities provide (see Chapter 8). The relationships between geography and structuring as well as the role played by organizational size are discussed at the end of the chapter.

Matrix Organizations

Matrix organizations are simultaneous combinations of functional and divisional arrangements; they are much like large cross-functional teams. A pure matrix organization can have two or more leaders over a single area—one from a functional area, like engineering, and the other from a product or geographic division. Realistically, however, most matrix structures do not represent equal divisions of authority. Few give equal authority to both dimensions of the matrix. One leader (often the divisional manager) is usually dominant in such key areas as budgeting, personnel reporting and appraisal, and strategy formulation.

Matrix structures, nevertheless, often improve the information distribution across an organization's functional or divisional units. In a matrix structure, functional personnel have designated roles and organizationally are required to interact and coordinate with product managers. This interchange can potentially reduce development times and time to market. Accordingly, matrix structures are often introduced in situations where integration can provide competitive advantages, such as in vertically and horizontally integrated organizations. Because of this, matrix structures have been successful in drug manufacturing, aerospace, and automobile industries. Also, the matrix structure can be essential in the healthcare industry, where the possibilities for coordination across multiple units, especially when they are geographically proximate, are great.

Like all structural arrangements do, matrix organizations present a number of problems. First, having two bosses can prevent the development of congruent goals and can increase power struggles. Second, units might develop group-itis, a feeling that all decisions need to be made by consensus. Third, functional specialists may lose touch with their specialty unit and become more product oriented. Fourth, matrix organizations can become overly complex, resulting in too many head office staffs to administer the complicated systems. This formalization can cause greater inflexibility that can be detrimental to innovation and strategic maneuvering. In fact, Peters and Waterman (1982, 76) state that a matrix organization "virtually always ceases to be innovative, often after just a short time.... It also regularly degenerates into anarchy and rapidly becomes bureaucratic and non-creative."

Healthcare organizations need to monitor the value of their structures and change as needed to more fully engage their strategies. Burns and Wholey (1993) found that almost one-fourth of all large teaching hospitals had adopted matrix structures by 1978 and that these adoptions were influenced by both the complexity of their services and external pressures. In addition, most hospitals, after adopting such structures, tended to retain them and did not transition into other structural forms. Such unwillingness to change might indicate the slide into a more bureaucratic and noncreative structure.

Some form of matrix structure is likely needed in situations where integration is a major objective. Some hospitals have attempted to solve the limitations of matrix structures by entering into mergers, thereby attempting to eliminate the organizational walls that separate the otherwise independent entities. The merger between the two HCA hospitals in Richmond (discussed in Chapter 6) is an example of this tactic. By merging their two south-side hospitals, HCA was able to move much more rapidly toward the integration not just of administrative functions but of clinical services as well. Such mergers can eliminate the necessity for adopting the complex matrix structures, which can mushroom out of control, while leaving in place preexisting structural divisions.

Virtual Organizations

Another structural form—the virtual organization—needs to be mentioned, principally because so many provider organizations attempted it in the 1990s. Although widely utilized outside of healthcare, the *virtual organization* has not always been successful.

The virtual organization is an interorganizational collaboration that does not involve common or full ownership (Barringer and Harrison 2000; Das and Teng 2000; Doz and Hamel 1998; Dussauge and Garrette 1999; Lorange and Roos 1991; Mol 2001). These arrangements are known by many names, including alliances, partnerships, joint ventures, networks, consortia, trade associations, loose coupling, and interlocking directorates. In this structural form, organizations are brought together through contracts and other exchange agreements to accomplish usually minor multiorganizational objectives (Miles and Snow 1992). In the healthcare industry, however, virtual organizational structures have been used to accomplish highly important strategic objectives; this use has been the source of many problems associated with this organizational form.

Virtual organizations are created through formal agreements between two or more organizations to pursue a set of common goals through the sharing of resources (e.g., intellectual property, people, capital, organizational capabilities, physical assets) and decision-making processes. The motivations for creating virtual organizations range from purely economic (e.g., searching for economies of scale, developing new technologies, joint purchasing of supplies, developing capital, risk sharing) to political (e.g., lobbying) to strategic (e.g., building market power, joint contracting with insurers). Such combinations might also be attempted when growth is constrained by market barriers such as legal constraints, access to distribution channels, established customer loyalty, lack of capital, and high costs.

Nonownership relationships are ideal in highly uncertain situations in which flexibility to enter or withdraw from a relationship is needed. Virtual relationships not only involve less investment on the front end, they are more reversible as well. The flip side of this is that partners to such ventures, because their commitments are less, cannot be relied on to remain in a strained relationship. In fact, such possibilities undermined a number of virtual arrangements established by healthcare providers in the 1990s. The Jacksonville merger of hospitals belonging to the Daughters of Charity and the Baptist Health System (mentioned in Chapter 7) is a variation of a virtual organizational structure. Called an operational merger, the two sponsoring organizations retained ownership of the physical facilities and the right to withdraw, should the need for such arise. When the much-anticipated threats from managed care and Columbia/HCA did not materialize, ongoing internal conflicts and incompatibilities eventually overwhelmed the weak structural mechanisms binding the two organizations, resulting in the dismantling of the operational merger.

Such weaknesses highlight the need for organizations that utilize virtual ventures to invest the requisite capital and build management capacity. Failure to do this is a primary reason that many such structures do not succeed. The challenges inherent in making them work are even greater when they are used to accomplish significant strategic purposes. This is illustrated in the virtual firm, discussed below.

The Virtual Firm

In the 1990s, many healthcare providers adopted virtual structures to accomplish some important strategic objectives. The use of such structures often reflected these providers' desire to retain autonomy while responding to rapidly changing environmental and market forces. In addition, employment of the virtual approach illustrated a widespread wariness to a complete merger or acquisition. Those that adopted this structural form unwittingly participated in a significant and somewhat unrealistic real-world experiment with structure-strategy combinations.

In their typology of structure-strategy combinations, displayed in Figure 10.1, Luke, Begun, and Pointer (1989) contrasted ownership-based ventures against virtual organizations in terms of the degree to which each form pursued limited and significant strategic purposes. As shown in the figure, organizations with tight ownership structures fall into two categories, depending on the level of strategic purpose. Those for which the strategic purpose is limited are referred to as "latent firms," and those for which the purpose is significant (e.g., to dominate markets, countervail buyers) are labeled simply as "firms." An example of latent firms is a cluster of public hospitals such as the Harris County Hospital District in Houston, which serves fairly well defined and noncompetitive market segments. Choice of the term "latent" suggests that although an organization might not currently be actively engaged in competitive combat, in time the organization can evolve into having a more aggressive strategic orientation, depending on changes in policy, market forces, and the environment.

Organizations that rely on loose structures also can be classified in two categories: those that have fairly limited strategic purposes are labeled "joint ventures," and those for which the combination is highly important strategically are referred to as "virtual firms." Here, the word "firm"

Figure 10.1. Virtual Firm: A Unique Organizational Form

Ownership Arrangement

Tight Structure   Loose Structure

		Tight Structure	Loose Structure
Strategic Purpose	*Significant*	Firms	**Virtual Firms**
	Limited	Latent Firms	Joint Ventures

Source: Adapted from Luke, R., J. Begun, and D. Pointer. 1989. "Quasi-Firms: Strategic Interorganizational Forms in the Health Care Industry." The *Academy of Management Review* 14 (1): 1–14. Used with permission.

connotes the high strategic purpose shared by the coventuring organizations. The partnership between two hospitals to provide management support to a third hospital (such as the Carilion–Centra Health collaborative effort discussed in Chapter 5) is an example of a joint venture. This organizational form typically requires from the partner organizations minimal overall operational or strategic commitments and compromises. The *virtual firm* category is especially unique to healthcare. In the 1990s, a number of provider organizations used loose structures to accomplish what would ordinarily be done through ownership arrangements—that is, mergers or acquisitions. These organizations formed major rival organizations that competed directly and generally within their local markets. The use of loose arrangements, however, loaded a heavy strategic weight onto relatively fragile organizational frames. As a result, many of these arrangements either failed in a few short years or evolved into more tightly structured arrangements.

The hospital sector has seen a number of virtual firms that made sufficient structural adjustments to facilitate their high strategic objectives while sustaining the virtual model. For example, three virtual firms initiated in Denver, Colorado, in the 1990s not only remain intact but also have emerged as the leading players in that highly competitive market. These organizations are (1) the Centura Health System, which combines facilities otherwise operated by Catholic Health Initiatives with hospitals owned by PorterCare Adventist Health System; (2) HealthOne, which combines the Denver-based HCA hospitals with a local not-for-profit hospital cluster; and (3) Exempla Health, the combination of Saint Joseph Hospital (owned by Sisters of Charity) and Lutheran Medical

Center. HealthOne, which started out as a 50/50 partnership, is now effectively run and controlled by the more dominant partner, HCA. Centura has strengthened its central leadership structure, significantly overcoming many of the limitations of loosely structured organizational forms (see Strategy Note 10.1). Notably, even with their reliance on relatively looser organizational structures, these three systems together control just around 79 percent of the acute care market in Denver.

The Promina Health System in Atlanta, Georgia, is another example of a virtual firm that has survived by tightening its otherwise loosely coupled organizational structures. Formed in 1994, Promina currently combines three smaller health systems, any one of which can withdraw from the alliance but at some cost. Corporate has the authority to approve hospital budgets, appoint hospital CEOs, and approve strategic plans, among other important powers. On the other hand, Promina (which initially comprised four systems), has lost some members, including the two-hospital Piedmont Hospital System, which in 2003 announced its intention to withdraw from Promina. This highlights the limitations inherent in utilizing loose structures to accomplish high strategic ends.

Finally, a number of very large and highly prominent Catholic hospital systems have adopted the virtual firm structure: Ascension Health, Catholic Healthcare Partners, Catholic Healthcare West, Catholic Health East, and Catholic Health Initiatives. These systems have survived only by turning over to the corporate center important operational and strategic powers. In most such combinations, the collaborating Catholic orders retain ownership of the physical facilities, but they have delegated most operational and strategic decision making to the corporate heads; as a result, this enables the systems to operate as if they were "firms."

STRATEGY AS A DETERMINANT OF STRUCTURE

In this section, we identify which of the three major structural forms—functional, divisional, and matrix—might best accommodate the company-level horizontal expansion types discussed in Chapter 8. Recall that the key dimensions are the size of the system and the geographic configuration of the system's facilities. Geographic configuration reflects the relative dispersion of the system's facilities—low and high).

Figure 10.2 illustrates the likely structural forms expected for system size and geographic configuration. In general, as organizations expand from small to large or from tightly configured to dispersed, they are expected to move from functional to divisional structures. Divisional

Figure 10.2. Strategy-Structure Relationship for Horizontally Expanded Hospital Systems

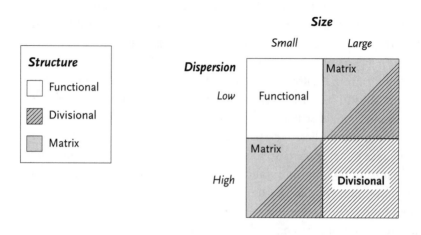

structures accommodate the increasing complexities associated with increasing scale and dispersion. In those "in between" situations, in which organizations are either small and dispersed or large and tightly configured, some variation on the matrix model (which combines elements from both functional and divisional structures) might be needed. Matrix structures might benefit large, tightly configured systems, such as Sutter Health in California, by helping them capture the benefits of both large size (for which divisional structures might be ideal) and high integrative potential associated with low dispersion (for which functional structures might work best).

The particular structural form needed to manage a multihospital organization might be fairly obvious. For example, Bon Secours Health System, which is spread up and down the East Coast, is an unmistakable candidate for a geographic-based divisional structure because of the great distances that separate most of its facilities. Bon Secours's five hospitals located in the New York and New Jersey area would not likely be very interdependent with its six hospitals in Virginia. In fact, Bon Secours is organized geographically into local systems, mostly divided by state: the system has facilities in nine states. Because of the uniqueness and particular challenges of the Virginia markets, Bon Secours has established separate organizational subunits in Norfolk and Richmond.

In other cases, the appropriate structural form might not be so obvious. MedStar Health (a relatively small multimarket system that has facilities in Baltimore, Maryland, and nearby Washington, DC) might need a divisional structure to accommodate the distinctive demands of its two very different markets. On the other hand, because the two markets are highly interdependent in terms of patient flows, referral patterns, insurers, and buyers, MedStar might need to adopt either a product-based divisional structure or possibly a functional structure. Given geographic proximities and the resultant potential for integration, matrix structures might also be needed to maximize the potential of this tightly clustered system.

Other Determinants of Structure

A number of other factors influence the choice of organizational structure, including factors that are both external and internal to organizations.

External Factors

From a strategic point of view, the structure of the market often plays a key role in shaping an organization's structure. A competitor that operates in markets composed of relatively equal and highly powerful oligopoly competitors might need a more adaptive structure to facilitate rapid responses to the moves of rivals. By contrast, a competitor that operates in small urban markets or rural communities, because it would generally face limited competitive threat, might adopt relatively more functional centralization to the corporate level.

In general, the relative stability of markets or of the broader environment is an especially important determinant of organizational structure. External stability allows an organization to refine existing processes and minimize the search for new information and discovery. Under such conditions, existing knowledge and skills are relatively easily obtained and preserved; functional centralization is thus more appropriately applied under such conditions. Multimarket hospital systems, for example, might want to centralize a number of functions during periods when the local markets are relatively stable, even while retaining a divisional structure. By contrast, unstable environments increase the need for information; adaptive capability; and, consequently, greater decentralization. Significant uncertainty, for example, was created in the 1990s when managed care companies moved rapidly to penetrate markets and engaged in aggressive

Table 10.1. Uncertainty and the Centralization of Decision Making

Locus of Decision Making

		Centralized	Decentralized
Locus of Uncertainty	*Individual Market*		√
	Industry/General Environment	√	

efforts to consolidate their markets. This forced hospitals, physicians, even supply companies to consider changes not only in their strategies but in their organizational structures as well.

On the other hand, how functional activities and decision making are structured will depend significantly on the locus of uncertainty. As indicated in Table 10.1, if the uncertainty originates uniquely within individual markets, then strategic functions and decision making might need to be decentralized to that level. If, however, the uncertainty is more generalized—say, at the level of the industry or general economy—then centralization might be the more appropriate response.

Internal Factors

A number of internal factors also affect the choice of structure and organizational strategy. The organization's product type, processes, types of interaction, organizational facilitation capability, and other factors influence the choice of organizational structure. Standardization, well-understood processes, low intensity of interaction, and available economies of scale can facilitate the use of more centralized structures. Products that are naturally standardized require less customization; their inputs and outputs can be more homogeneous, thus allowing for more formalized practices and operating procedures. McDonalds, the fast-food chain, exemplifies this concept. That company's inputs and outputs are highly prescribed and consistent across the world. The process of making french fries, including the purchasing and frying of potatoes, meets rigorous prewritten standards. As a result, McDonalds' fries taste relatively the same at almost any of their restaurants worldwide. By contrast, the software industry might face much more diversity and customization across markets and clients, requiring greater flexibility by client, product, and location that can be facilitated by a multidivisional structure.

Some healthcare products lend themselves more readily to standardization. An obstetric service for normal deliveries or surgery for a common ailment can be viewed as much more standardized, at least when compared to psychiatric service and internal medicine. Nonclinical, back-office services (such as billing and admissions) and support services (such as dietary and housekeeping) are also more easily standardized and can be preprogrammed by organizational policy. Greater standardization, and greater centralization, can thus be expected in back office and support services as well as (to a somewhat lesser degree) in clinical services such as obstetrics and surgery. Also, those multihospital systems that operate in relatively "standardized" small general hospitals, mostly in nonurban markets (i.e., Community Health Systems, Health Management Associates, LifePoint, Province Healthcare, and Triad) might combine functional and divisional structures. They are likely to centralize as many tasks as is practicable and delegate to regional division heads responsibility for implementing corporate decisions and budgetary expectations.

The intensity of interaction has also been a factor in the optimal selection of organizational structure. Lawrence and Lorsch (1967) divided levels of interaction into pooled, sequential, and reciprocal. Processes that involve pooled interactions are easily segmented, such that figurative walls can be drawn around specific processes. Lawrence and Lorsch used as an example a bank's branches, which share common functions and have pooled interests (e.g., positioning, shared investment activities) but otherwise remain relatively autonomous in terms of their service to specific markets and customer segments. (Since Lawrence and Lorsch wrote their influential book, *Organization and Environment*, a majority of banks have merged and experienced substantial changes to the point that many banking transactions have been centralized and converted to more sequential or reciprocal processes.) Horizontally expanded multihospital systems that have facilities dispersed widely across the country exhibit pooled interactions in selected functions. For example, HCA's hospitals and local clusters are clinically autonomous, but they share common identifiers, finances, and administrative policies and systems, regionally and nationally.

Organizations that have sequential interactions, on the other hand, pass their products or customers from one part of the organization to another in a sequential fashion. This assembly line process involves greater interactions than is experienced between pooled processes. In healthcare, sequential processes often occur between departments, such as between admissions, patient care, and service support as well as between facilities and

HEALTHCARE STRATEGY

individual providers. Sequential processes are explicitly assumed to exist in the clinical pathways and protocols being developed and used in hospitals (Walston and Bogue 1999). Much of acute care, especially the highly complex and technical services, involve extensive sequential interactions. Intensive care patients, for example, have multiple, repeated, intense interactions with physicians, nurses, and other ancillary personnel. Vertically integrated organizations must structure their sequential interactions as well. All such intense interactions work best under decentralized decision-making structures. Processes involving less interaction invite more centralized decision making because fewer adjustments are needed.

CONCLUSION

A key to gaining competitive advantage is the ability to make timely, informed, and quality decisions. Choosing the right balance among the available structural forms—functional, divisional, and matrix—can make such an important difference in the success with which strategy is formulated and implemented. Leaders of healthcare organizations, who are involved in forming more complex multiorganizational forms, especially need to understand the relationship between organizational growth and organizational structuring.

The virtual organization, which became fashionable in the industry in the 1990s, needs to be evaluated carefully in terms of the degree to which nonownership-based arrangements are capable of supporting the implementation of major strategic objectives. Although the thought that important strategic moves can be accomplished without organizations having to give up long-cherished autonomies is attractive, sustainable competitive advantage might not be achievable with loose organizational structures. Some virtual alliances have succeeded over the last few years, but most of them have had to ensure that sufficient powers are turned over to the alliance headquarters to accomplish the requisite strategic adaptability and stability.

In sum, the strategy analyst must understand that choices about structure cannot be formularized. Rather, structures are highly contingent on many internal and external factors, not the least of which is strategy itself.

REFERENCES

Barringer, B. R., and J. S. Harrison. 2000. "Walking a Tightrope: Creating Value Through Interorganizational Alliances." *Journal of Management* 26: 367–403.

Burns, L., and D. Wholey. 1993. "Adoption and Abandonment of Matrix Management Programs: Effects of Organizational Characteristics and Interorganizational Networks." *Academy of Management Journal* 36 (1): 106–38.

Chandler, A. D. 1962. *Strategy and Structure: Chapters in the History of the Industrial Enterprise.* Cambridge, MA: MIT Press.

Das, T. K., and B. S. Teng. 2000. "Instabilities of Strategic Alliances: An Internal Tensions Perspective." *Organization Science* 11 (1): 77–106.

Doz, Y., and G. Hamel. 1998. *Alliance Advantage: The Art of Creating Value Through Partnering.* Boston: Harvard Business School Press.

Dussauge, P., and B. Garrette. 1999. *Cooperative Strategy: Competing Successfully Through Strategic Alliances.* New York: John Wiley & Sons.

Hammer, M., and J. Champy. 1993. *Reengineering the Corporation.* New York: Harper Collins.

Jones, A. 1987. *The Art of War in the Western World.* New York: Oxford University Press.

Lathrop, P. 1993. *Restructuring Health Care: The Patient Focused Paradigm.* San Francisco: Jossey-Bass.

Lawrence, P., and J. Lorsch. 1967. *Organization and Environment.* Boston: Harvard Business School Press.

Lorange, P., and J. Roos. 1991. "Why Some Strategic Alliances Succeed and Others Fail." *Journal of Business Strategy* 12 (1): 25–30.

Luke, R., J. Begun, and D. Pointer. 1989. "Quasi-Firms: Strategic Interorganizational Forms in the Health Care Industry." *The Academy of Management Review* 14 (1): 1–14.

Miles, R., and C. Snow. 1992. "Causes of Failure in Network Organizations." *California Management Review* 34 (4): 53–65.

Mintzberg, H. 1994. *The Rise and Fall of Strategic Planning: Reconceiving Roles for Planning, Plans, Planners.* New York: The Free Press.

Mol, M. J. 2001. "Creating Wealth Through Working with Others: Interorganizational Relationships." *The Academy of Management Executive* 15 (1): 150–52.

Peters, T., and R. Waterman. 1982. *In Search of Excellence: Lessons from America's Best-Run Companies.* New York: Harper & Row.

Porter, M. E. 1985. *Competitive Advantage.* New York: The Free Press.

Rumelt, R. P. 1974. *Strategy, Structure, and Economic Performance.* Boston: Harvard Business School Press.

Smith, A. 1910. *The Wealth of Nations.* London: JM Dent & Sons.

Walston, S., and J. R. Kimberly. 1997. "Reengineering Hospitals: Experience and Analysis from the Field" *Hospital & Health Services Administration* 42: 143–63.

Walston, S., and R. Bogue. 1999. "The Effects of Reengineering: Fad or Competitive Factor?" *Journal of Healthcare Management* 44 (6): 456–76.

Williamson, O. 1975. *Markets and Hierarchies*. New York: The Free Press.

Index

About the Authors

ROICE D. LUKE, PH.D., is professor in the Department of Health Administration at the Virginia Commonwealth University (VCU) in Richmond, Virginia. He earned his BS and MBA degrees from the University of California at Berkeley and his PH.D. degree in medical care organization, with a cognate in health economics, from the University of Michigan, Ann Arbor. Prior to coming to VCU, Dr. Luke served on the faculty and as director of the health administration program at the University of Colorado at Denver. Also, he served as chair of the VCU department in the 1980s.

In addition, Dr. Luke has served as editor-in-chief of *Medical Care Review* and on the editorial boards of *Inquiry* and *Frontiers of Health Services Management*. An avid student of healthcare markets, Dr. Luke has maintained a unique and national database on local markets and systems since the late 1980s. In the 1990s, he directed a federally funded study of the performance of strategic hospital alliances and a six-year study of local markets and systems, which was funded by four major supply and distribution companies. He can be reached via e-mail at luker@hsc.vcu.edu.

STEPHEN L. WALSTON, PH.D., is an associate professor at Indiana University. He has served as the director of Indiana University's Master in Health Administration Program. Prior to his present position, he taught at Cornell University in Ithaca, New York. He earned BS and MPA degrees from Brigham Young University in Provo, Utah, and a PH.D. from the University of Pennsylvania's Wharton School, completing the requirements of the school's Health Care Systems Department and Management Department. Prior to returning for his doctoral degree, Dr. Walston worked in healthcare administration for 14 years, the last 10 of which were spent as a chief executive officer for hospitals in the western United States.

Dr. Walston's research explores organizational restructuring and the effects of new structures and processes on efficiency and effectiveness. He has done extensive work on reengineering and organizational effectiveness. His publications have appeared in many journals and books. He can be reached via e-mail at swalston@iupui.edu.

PATRICK MICHAEL PLUMMER is the founder and chief executive officer of myHealthcareNews.com, the largest news-aggregating service for the business of healthcare on the Internet. Before starting myHealthcare News.com in 2003, Mr. Plummer founded U.S. LifeLine, Inc., a company that focused exclusively on healthcare group purchasing organizations (GPOs). At USL, Mr. Plummer was publisher and editor of *Major Account News* and *The Health Strategist*, two of the most highly respected senior-level newsletters, and The MAX online database, which focused exclusively on the business of healthcare. Plummer sold USL in March 2000 to Neoforma, a healthcare business-to-business e-commerce company. Before starting U.S. LifeLine, Mr. Plummer served as vice president of AmeriNet and as product manager for Voluntary Hospitals of America. In addition, he has served at a Daughters of Charity hospital and a multihospital system as a biomedical engineer; has evaluated and recommended medical technologies as an M.D. buyline consultant; and has worked for SpaceLabs Medical, a manufacturer of patient-monitoring equipment.

Mr. Plummer is a frequent guest speaker at national and regional meetings. His knowledge and views regarding healthcare business strategy, market analysis, and group purchasing have been published multiple times. Mr. Plummer holds an MBA in management from Amber University and a BS in biomedical electronics from Thomas Edison State College. He can be reached via e-mail at patrick@myHealthcareNews.com.